Bad Nerves: Living with MS

By LJ Thomas

Printed in the United States of America

ISBN: 978-0-9970087-1-5

Published by Asoral Publishing

Over Design by LJ Thomas
Layout design by LJ Thomas
Back graphic by Freepik

Also by LJ Thomas
Tales of Survival: Domestic Violence
Children's series Leo Learns About Anger

Published under the pseudonym Jamela
What Is This World coming To? New Collection

Dedication

This book is dedicated to all of the persons living with Multiple Sclerosis and who try to explain the disease to others. I realize it is difficult to understand. I dedicate this book to all of the physicians, nurses, caregivers, families and friends who help take care of us. This book is also dedicated to the classmates and friends of my children through the years, who understood my limitations and did not mind being around me. I dedicate this book to my children for struggling to explain to others, what was wrong with their mother at the young ages of 6 and 4. I dedicate this book to my grandson, so that it will be easier for him to explain (though I don't think he's going to have a problem....lol).

Acknowledgements

I want to thank Jehovah for giving me the strength and presence of mind to write this book. Thank you to my husband, Carl and my daughters, Jasmine and Marilyn (Chris). Thank you to my parents for understanding when I first became sick. Thank you to my siblings for their support. Thank you to Dr. DeMichele (no longer with us) and Dr. Thrower for treating me and helping me to realize things about myself. I want to thank Dr. Renee' Watson and Krista Kozacki for realizing what was wrong and developing the necessary treatment plan. I want to thank Aunt Illa and Uncle Andy for helping to take care of my family when I could not even take care of myself. Thank you, Tami for coming to the house and helping with the girls and spending time with them. It really helped to distract them from having a sick mother. I want to acknowledge, Vanessa, Betty, Teake, Debbie, Sonya, Cathy and Jennifer for putting up with me, fussing at me and helping me realize when I was/am going overboard. I also want to acknowledge my grandma Cat, Neal and Lula. All three women were/are wise and gave me good advice throughout the time I've had/have with them. I appreciate my congregation for encouraging me and helping me. You have no idea how encouraging your words are to me and how loved you make me feel. Thank you to all of my "children" for helping to take care of me. Thank you Selena Walton for your input and suggestions.

Table of Contents

Daily Life with MS

Spring: A Typical Good Day

I can hear the birds chirping. As I look out the window, I can see the dogwood tree in the yard. It's fuzzy, but I can see it. Then it hits me. I begin to rub my nose profusely, try to scratch the inside of my ear and rub my eyes. I am having a hard time dealing with seasonal allergies. This is a daily occurrence. Once I am able to breathe, I try to stand up. So from the time I opened my eyes to the time I actually try to get out of bed is about 10-15 minutes. My poor husband listens to this and rarely says anything. He is fortunate enough not to have seasonal allergies. Trying to clear my nasal passages is a bother.

Today is a good day because I can actually see the tree in the yard. Yesterday, that was not the case. So, I try to swing my legs to the floor. Hmmm. I'm telling them to move, but they aren't listening. So, it's going to be one of those days. Okay. Since I am already in a sitting position, I prop the pillows up behind me. I reach over to the nightstand and grab the TV remotes.

Within the next 15 minutes, my husband comes into the room. "Get up lazy bum." he says jokingly.

"I am up. It's a bedroom day. The legs aren't working." I reply.

1

"Okay. Do you want to go to the bathroom now or do you want to use the potty?"

"I want to try to go to the bathroom. Besides, I want to go ahead and wash up. While I'm in the bathroom, will you put the bench in front of the sink for me, please?" I ask.

"Sure." He walks around to my side of the bed which is closest to the bathroom. All I have to do is get around the corner and the door to the bathroom is right there. It is not a long distance. He leans down and I follow our routine. I reach up and put my arms around his neck. But I decide to do something different.

"Let me try this. I'm going to scoot to the end of the bed and that should make it easier, plus it won't be so hard on your back." I suggest.

"Okay. I'll stand here and watch to make sure everything is okay." He says and steps back. I really love the fact that he lets me try things on my own before he tries to help. He allows me to have some level of independence.

It takes me a few minutes because I have to physically move my legs with my hands, but I finally make it to the foot of the bed, where is he standing. "Good girl. You are tired, aren't you?"

"Yes, but… I… don't….want… to… use the potty, I want to use the toilet." I say out of breath.

"Okay, can you sit and rest for a minute? I'm going to go check on this file and then I'll be right back." He says when I nod my head in the affirmative.

As I sit on the bed, I plan, how I will get to the bathroom and then the sink. I know that it is a short distance and pivoting will take a lot of the work out of it. True to his word, my Carl comes in the room, "Are you ready?"

"Yup. Let's do this!" I say with excitement

He walks over to me and leans forward. I suggest that he turn his back to me once I'm up and then as he walks my legs will drag behind. He does this and backs me into the bathroom and I sit on the toilet.

"Thank you. I'll yell for you when I'm ready to get washed up."

"What? You don't want me to see you or something?"

"Exactly. Now, get out. I need privacy, Sir." I respond jokingly.

"Fine, don't call me when you fall in." he says as he walks out of the room.

I'm left alone and I begin to think of the best way to get to the sink. I realize that he can get me there the same way and once seated on the shower bench, I can turn myself around. It will take some doing, but I can do it. Then I can bathe myself and once done he can help me get back into bed.

While sitting there, I make a mental 'to do list'. I have to get my laptop to put this in my journal. I need to remind him to take something out for dinner. Have Carl bring me the phone so I can call the people about the heat and the bills. Make a doctor's appointment. Call my friend and let her know that if my legs don't decide to work, that we won't be going to the meeting tonight and I'll have to see what tomorrow brings. I also need to remind Carl to go ahead and start the laundry. Once the clothes are dried, if he brings them to me, I can go ahead and fold them and he can hang the things that need hanging. If he puts the hangers on the bed, I can put them on the hangers, he'll just have to place them in the closet.

When I'm done, I yell, "Carl! I'm done!"

Within a few minutes, he walks into the room. "Oh, it's okay to see you now, huh?"

"Yup. Can you look in the top drawer and get me a clean pair of underwear and a bra, please. I'll call you again when I'm done."

"Okay. Are you sure? As a matter of fact, I'm going to sit here and watch TV while you bathe and I'll turn my back, so I can't see you." he says sarcastically.

"Okay, and you better not peak!" I say playfully.

He gets the items I ask for and places them on the vanity counter next to the sink. I reach beneath the counter and grab my toiletries (shower gel, toothpaste and baby oil). I use my hands to turn my legs around so I can face the counter. This makes it easier for me to reach the sink. Once I finish bathing, I say, "Okay, Carl, I'm ready."

He walks over and leans down so I can put my arms around his neck. Then once I am standing he turns around so that I am leaning on his back and he backs me up to the bed. I sit on the foot of the bed and scoot myself up to the head of the bed where I get under the covers using my hands to maneuver my legs. I am so tired when I'm done.

"I know you have some things that you want to take care of, but rest for a while first. That took a lot out of you. Tell me what you want me to do."

So I remind him to take something out for dinner, start the laundry and bring me my laptop and the phone. Since he wants to make sure I rest, he leaves to handle the first two assignments and doesn't bring the phone or my laptop until he returns. I hate when he does that. But, I understand. He says that I'm 'stubborn'. I say I'm 'strong willed and independent'.

The rest of the day progresses along slowly since I am confined to the bed. Things that I would normally do, I have to wait for someone to do them for me. As on I put clothes on hangers I sit in the bed, I exercise my legs as much as I can and pray that the movement will come back. If it doesn't, then I'll call the doc in a couple of days for an appointment.

Okay, my movement did not return, so I have spent the day sitting up in bed. I folded a couple loads of laundry and placed clothes on hangers for Carl to put in the closet. Most were his shirts anyway. Maybe tomorrow will be a better day.

A New Day

So, yesterday, I woke up and had no movement in my legs. Today is a new day. I open my eyes and I can see clearly. That is a good start. I can wiggle my toes. Another good sign. I stretch and I can move my legs. Yay! I'm back. I sit on the side of the bed and reach over to get my laptop as I am rubbing my nose and eyes, trying to breathe. Finally, I am finished with my morning nasal congestion and can focus on my plans for the rest of the day. Since Carl and I did the laundry yesterday, all I really have to do is some light cleaning and cook dinner. But, I want to be careful because I'm already tired and I just woke up. My legs feel like they weigh 50lbs each. My left arm is tingling and my back feels like someone has been punching me for hours. At least I can see clearly with both eyes today. Yesterday, I could see, but not clearly. Things were fuzzy.

I know that because I am past exhausted that I have to pace myself. I decided to sit up and take care of sitting tasks first, then go get something to eat. By then, it should be after 11am and I can hold it down. I hate that my stomach does that and I have to wait so long before I can eat anything. That is, if I want to keep it inside my body so that I can digest it. Anyway, Carl hears me moving and comes into the room. "How do you feel? You didn't sleep well last night."

"I'm sorry if I disturbed you." I comment apologetically.

"No, it's okay. I could tell you were in pain because you moaned and tossed and turned all night. So, I want you to get some rest today. Take it easy, LaRosa. I mean it. What do you want to eat?"

"In a few minutes, can you bring me some cereal? The legs are working today, so I can get to the bathroom on my own. I'm not going to take a shower, just do a bird bath because I'm exhausted and I don't want to risk falling again. See, I'm trying to be safe and smart about things." I say with a huge smile.

He leaves the room and a few minutes later he comes in with the cereal. I have already gone to the bathroom and am about to bathe. I sit and eat the cereal, although it's a little too early. But since he went through the trouble to get it for me, I go ahead and eat it. I don't want him to think I'm ungrateful. Besides, I need to rest for a minute and this gives me a break without looking like I'm taking a break. Once I'm done with the food, I find something to wear and bathe. I sit and rest for a few minutes before gathering the breakfast dishes and leaving the room.

When I walk into the living room, he is watching TV. The studio light is on, so I know he is back and forth. I take a closer look and realize that he is reviewing a video that was done when the kids were small. "Hey, I haven't seen that in years."

"Yeah. I found this and some other tapes and decided that I'm doing to put them on DVD. I was just going through them. The quality on DVD is so much better and no one uses VHS anymore. Plus it will be easier to store them. Do you have any blank DVD's?" he inquires.

"Yup. If you look in the bottom drawer of my night stand, there is a brand new spindle of DVD's. You can open it and get a few. Leave me some because I have to get all this music off my system to make room for some other things."

"Oh, so you've been holding out on me, huh?"

"No, I just got them a few days ago when I went to the store. If you had gone with me, I would have bought you a spindle, but since you didn't I only got one for me. I did not know you needed DVD's."

"Yeah, right. Whatever Rosie, whatever." Came is playful reply

I sit down for a few minutes and it turns into hours. When I realize what time it is, it is after noon. I still have to take something out for dinner. Jasmine and Marilyn will be coming home soon and I know they'll be hungry. Just then, my cell phone buzzes. It is Jasmine saying that she wants pizza and that they are ordering the pizza to be delivered. She also says that they are leaving work early and want to know if Carl can come pick them up in an hour. I relay the message and continue to rest. He leaves to get the girls within about 45 minutes since we do not live far from their job at Six Flags. When he leaves, I go into the kitchen to get the paper plates for the pizza. I don't feel like washing any dishes and I know the girls won't either. Carl rarely washes dishes, so paper is the way to go.

After we eat, the girls clean the kitchen and I slowly make my way back to my bedroom. Once I sit on the bed, I realize that I did not get any cleaning done and I basically sat around all day. Even though I rested, my legs still feel like they each weigh 50 lbs, my left arm is still tingling and my back is still killing me. I'm going to give it a few days and if I don't feel better, I'm going to have to see the doc, for sure. I do another bird bath, thinking that I will be able to take a shower in the morning and get into bed. I turn the TV to my favorite channel and the next thing I know, it is morning.

Summer: A typical day

I love the bright sunny days of summer. But, summer does not love me. This is what I mean. On an average day, once I can literally drag myself out of the bed, it is downhill from there. Why? Because I am trying to carry around weights for legs, I can barely see most days and I am constantly shifting my weight because of back pain. I wake up exhausted. I mean I wake up feeling like I've worked a 24 hour shift doing heavy manual labor. The exhaustion is so overwhelming that I barely have the energy to sit up sometimes. As a result, I spend a great deal of the season indoors and trying to get rest. Even when I sleep, Carl tells me that it is a restless sleep. He says that I toss and turn all night and that I'm always moaning in pain during the night. The ironic thing is that I take pain medication every night before going to bed. All in all, summer is beautiful to watch from my window. That is how I get to enjoy it.

Of course, I'm a little particular about buying my own groceries. Since I only shop at stores which are open all night, I get to buy my food sometimes. Since the humidity is so high during the summer months, I limit my time outside. As a result, when I am physically able, I go to the grocery store in the wee hours of the morning. Not only is it much cooler, but there are less crowds and I can take my time. I don't have to worry about hitting people who aren't paying attention since I use the motorized cart. My girls say that I am dangerous on the cart because I only blow the horn once. But, if I can hear people talking on the next aisle, then they should be able to hear a loud motorized cart coming and that's why I only beep the horn once. Since my life during the summer is so limited, I look forward to shopping for groceries. It's kind of sad. But that's my life.

Fall: A Typical Day

Now, I love the colors of the fall. I hate the rain. I hate the coolness on the air. I can feel my muscles starting to stiffen as the weather gets cooler. True, this is a welcome break from the humidity of the summer. I can leave the house if it not raining or too cool. This is also the season, where my allergies start to really act up. So, not only am I doing my normal nasal routine, but I'm dealing with stiffness and aches. What does this mean? Hmm. Let's see. Once I can actually get out of bed, and this is rare. I am bundled up in several layers of clothes. I tend to get cold easily, even with the central heat on and a small heater next to me. So, I crochet and this also helps keep me warm. I'm not very good at it, but it is something to do and gives me a sense of accomplishment.

Oftentimes, Carl is home with me. I used to think it was because he was a possessive man. But, then I realized it's because he wants to make sure I'm safe. He tries to find work that he can do from home so that he can stay with me. Apparently, I've had too many falls where I've hit my head. I know that I have vertigo and that is one explanation for the falls. But another is that my legs get weak and I the ground or floor. I try not to hit my head, but this cannot always be avoided. Hence, I have protective family members. I am thankful for them. They frequently notice things that I don't. Even though I challenge them on safety issues, I know they are doing it because they love me. It just makes me feel like I'm a child when my children and husband have to do simple things like get me something to eat. I should be doing that for them.

I don't drive because of the vertigo and other issues. Can I drive? I think so. But, they all say 'no'. Even my son-in-law. But I guess I should be happy that I have such a good support system. Many people do not have anything like this.

Now, what do I really like to do in the fall? Well, I enjoy taking warm to hot baths. The way the temperature of the water just melts away the stiffness is amazing. However, this is a catch 22. Why? If you'll remember, humidity causes me to become very fatigued. So, when I take a bath, I prepare to sit there for a long time. Of course, the rule in my house is that I cannot take a bath without someone else being home. Carl usually helps me into and out of the tub. He comes in to check on me, if I have not called out to him by the time he thinks I should. I always ask him to wash my back. Before I get in the tub, I generally turn some music on and try to sing while bathing. Ha ha ha, that's funny.

Once I finish bathing, Carl comes back and helps me out of the tub. I notice him watching how my legs move. Once I'm dried off and get to the bed, he usually tells me to sit there and that he'll be back in a few. Generally, I obey because I'm too exhausted to do anything else. So, this time serves to goals. I get to rest and it gives my body time to get itself together. Usually after about 30 minutes, I can get into bed. This takes so much out of me that I usually fall right to sleep. Carl often tells me that he comes back and I am asleep. Of course, he teases me about this, but that is to be expected. This is a typical day during the fall. What about winter?

Winter: An Average day

Well… this season it difficult, to say the least. I have the stiffness of the fall coupled with the allergies of the spring. In addition, it is cold which makes me hurt. What do I do? Spend most of my time indoors. There is no good and bad day during this season. I have pain medication, but I often choose not to take it. Why? Because I do not want to sleep my life away. So, I manage my pain psychologically. At least until it becomes so unbearable that I am forced to take something. I recently learned that pain is one of the goals that healthcare professionals try to alleviate since it causes stress on the body. As a result, I have been trying to minimize the amount of pain I am in. My girls always tell healthcare professionals (doctors, nurses and such) that I have a high tolerance for pain. I don't think so. If I did, I would never need pain meds. But, I do go days without taking anything and I'll just find a way to block it out of my mind. Is this the right thing to do? Nope. But, it works for me. I am working on not doing it but, it's hard.

Now, when I wake in the morning, even though the leaves are dead, my allergies still act up. So, the first thing I do is clear my nasal passages. Once this is done, I try to make my way to the bathroom. If I can successfully do this, then I let Carl know that I'm about to take a shower. Lately, I have been taking my shower at night and doing a bird bath in the morning. This helps me sleep. I often wake up at night and it takes a while for me to get back to sleep. It doesn't happen all the time, but when it does, it lasts for a few months. I hate lying there looking at my eyelids and hurting, while Carl is next to me sleeping like a baby. But, that is my life. Once I get dressed, I usually head to the kitchen to take something out for dinner. Since I am cold natured, I'm always careful to put on socks and house shoes, a long sleeved shirt or sweater and long pants. This way, I can be warm. Even with a small heater next to me and warm clothes, I still get extremely cold. Sometimes, I get into bed and get under the covers. When this happens, I generally have two quilted bedspreads and a doubled over quilt on my side of the bed. Poor Carl gets hot easily and he actually sleeps in the same bed with me like this. Anyone who walks into our bedroom can instantly tell which side of the bed belongs to me, if they really know me.

So, during the day, I take it easy. I do a little light cleaning, picking up things out of place and putting them away and fluffing the pillows. Since vacuuming causes pain, I don't do this. But, I am really particular about my kitchen. So, I always make sure the dishes are washed and put away. I make sure the stove and fridge are clean and free of food stains. I usually get one of the girls to mop the floor at least once a week. I wipe the hood and counters daily, because I hate any kind of buildup. Of course, Carl teases me and says that I have OCD. I may have this, but at least my kitchen is clean. If anyone comes to the house and they see that the kitchen is a mess, they know that I don't feel well or was too tired to clean anything.

During this time of year, it takes me a long time to cook. I generally start around 3pm to have the food ready by 6 or 6:30 that evening. I am moving slow because of the pain and stiffness. And my normally swift movements are gone. It's hard for me to think and I have to plan a lot more. In addition, since it takes so long to cook, I often make soups and meals in the slow cooker. When I cook on Sunday, I try to make enough to last for a few days. This is usually easier because the girls will help me cook. The things that I have trouble doing like cutting vegetables, they do for me. If I make something that requires mixing, they also do this. I like when we cook together because we get to spend time together and have fun joking around with each other. Once we eat dinner, the girls clean the kitchen. After a couple of hours watching TV, I go to my room to go to bed. Sometimes, I read or turn the TV on and let it watch me once I fall asleep. Even so, I know I'm going to wake up in the middle of the night. This is the worse time of year for me, because I feel like I have to have help with everything. I am dependent on everyone else to get things accomplished. I am a burden to everyone I know.

My Story: The Beginning

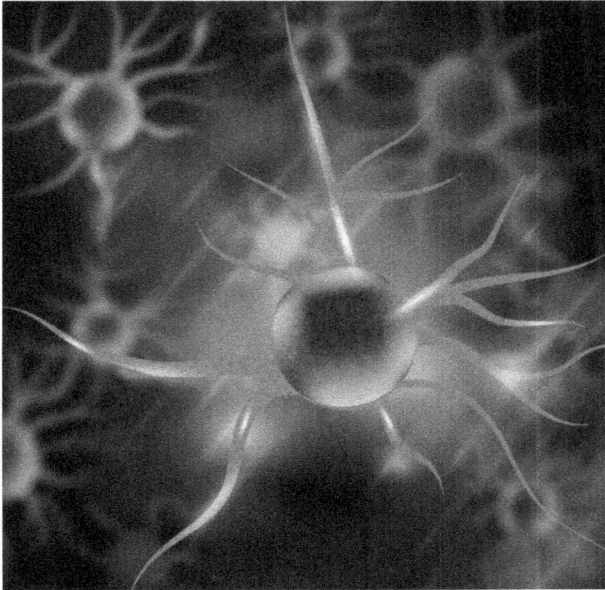

Ok, just to make sure things are clear; this is not a medical book and the information contained herein, should not be used as such. If you suspect that you or someone you know has Multiple Sclerosis (MS), please see a neurologist. This is information for people who have no idea what MS (Multiple Sclerosis) is and how people live with it. The accounts are true and show the wide variety of ways the disease manifests itself. MS is a terrible unpredictable disease. Please seek medical help if necessary.

So, what are 'bad nerves'? Don't worry about that right now. When I say 'bad nerves', I am not referring to nerves involved in criminal activities. I am referring to connections. Since there were so many persons who know little to nothing about MS, I began explaining my illness as 'bad nerves'. Let me give you some background on me and my diagnosis.

I am a 50 year-old African American mother of 30 and 28 year old daughters. I have been married 30 years. I was born in Baltimore, Maryland, but the family relocated back to Florence, South Carolina, where my parents met. I was never a child in the best of health. I've had asthma and allergies for as long as I can remember. I was raised in a small southern town. We relocated back to Baltimore in 1979 and stayed for three years. I hated living in the big city. The people were so violent. Needless to say, during our very first winter in Baltimore, I fell and had a terrible accident (country girl takes a tumble).

Here's how it happened. It snowed one day and then the snow melted. A couple of days later I was leaving the house to walk to school with a friend who would come by and picked me up every morning so we could walk together for safety. (It was a dangerous time, but I'll save that for another book.) My mother had purchased boots for me to wear in this kind of winter weather. Since I had never walked in snow before, I was extra careful as we left for school. Our apartment was on the ground floor, but it was at the top of about 10 brick steps. I walked cautiously across the porch and grabbed onto the railing to descend the steps. I stepped on the very first step and that was all I remembered for a while (a couple of days later things started coming back to me, plus my mother told me what happened). My head really hurt in the back on right side.

According to my mother, I slipped on a piece of ice and fell down the whole flight of stairs, hitting my head on each step as I traveled down my slippery slope. They tried to catch me, but it all happened so fast. She hurriedly put me in the car and rushed me to the nearest hospital. She said she asked me questions as she drove to the hospital since she was trying to keep me awake. According to her, I did not see white snow, it was red and that scared her. She said I was very sleepy and kept holding the back of my head and complaining of a headache. Once we were seen in the ER, a CT scan was done and my mother was advised to keep me home from school for a few days and not to let me sleep for a while. She was told that I had a pin-sized hole where I hit my head so many times. I was so tired and I could not remember what happened.

Needless to say after a few days I returned to school. It was so much harder than before my fall, but I figured it was because I had been out for a few days. I was 12 years old when the fall happened. By the time we moved back to South Carolina and I was 15 years, I was wearing glasses and suffering from migraines. Surprisingly, the first year of school in South Carolina was easy. They wanted to move me to the next grade (they did the same thing when we moved to Baltimore, but I refused both times. Imagine my surprise when they wanted to skip me after hearing all the stereotypes about people from the South being dumb). Nevertheless, school progressed along and things were normal in my teenage life, well as normal as they could be for me.

It turned out that I contracted "the kissing disease" during the last semester of my sophomore year. I was out with a dear friend one day and I was having a good time. It was fairly warm outside (April and May in South Carolina can be downright hot) and I was so tired. I felt like I would faint while she was talking to this lady about the Bible. Ironically, the woman was complaining that we could be spreading diseases. I managed to make it through the conversation and to the car. Once we got in the car.

My friend took me straight home. Once again, my mother rushed me to the doctor (ER). Imagine my surprise when the test results came back and the doctor said, "Oh, you have the kissing disease." He was so calm about it, like it was an everyday thing! Meanwhile, I was mortified and trying to figure out how to tell my mother that I had not been kissing anyone. He said a person could have it and not even know it. Needless to say I burst out, "Momma, I didn't kiss anybody. There is nobody that I want to kiss!" She looked at me with murder in her eyes so I knew I was going to get it when we got home. The doctor realized that I was scared to death of what my mother would do and explained the disease. He said the medical name is Mononucleosis (also called Epstein- Barr Virus) and it is called "the kissing disease' because it is so easy to catch. He said it is possible to get it through a cough. I was so happy the doctor explained that to my mother. To this day, I truly believe he saved my life. My mother was and still is a "no nonsense women", hence the fear for the loss of my life.

He also explained that I should get plenty of rest and fluids. I should not do a lot of jumping around (this wasn't a problem for me anyway since my favorite thing to do was read). He asked if I was taking PE (Physical Education) in school and when I told him that I would be taking it the next school year, he mentioned that I would need an excuse. Since persons with this disease are advised to avoid contact sports and strenuous physical activity, I would not be allowed to do those things in PE (Good, I thought, since I absolutely hated P.E. I guess that is to be expected when a person is athletically challenged).

I was working on a term paper for school on the subject of Anorexia Nervosa. My mother thought that I was not eating because of the term paper. She commented on how much weight I had lost and how I slept all the time. I tried to assure her that there was nothing wrong with me. But after the doctor gave his diagnosis, she felt better. As a result, my junior year of high school was easy. I went to PE and dressed out, but that was all. I did well on the written work and assisted the coach when he needed it. I spent a lot of time in the weight room using the equipment (I had strong legs as a result of leg pressing).

The rest of my high school years were not filled with medical uniqueness, thank goodness. I met my husband at 19 and by the age of 20, I was married and a mother. We relocated to Oxford Mississippi for us to go to school (and other familial reasons) in 1987. We moved back to South Carolina in 1988 because my asthma was horrible in Mississippi. By July of 1989 I had my second daughter (a difficult pregnancy). Life went along fairly normally for a while.

My husband worked a full time job and worked on his music career in the evenings and on the weekends. In 1992 I had a hysterectomy (boy was I happy!). I returned to work and found it difficult to do my job. My eyes were constantly running water and there was always a buildup of mucus (especially in the left eye). In addition, it was hard for me to see. Sometimes my vision was blurred and sometimes the vision was completely gone. Finally, I made an appointment to see the eye doctor for a new prescription for my glasses. I got the glasses and realized they weren't working. At the same time, I was having really bad headaches. I was making mistakes at work, but I did not want to talk to my boss about it (She was telling other people that she was paying me twice what I was actually being paid (This really upset me when I found out. She was complaining about me not wearing the latest fashions and going to the salon each week to get my hair done. She was constantly comparing me to the secretary before me who was single with no children. I found this behavior from her appalling since I was the Operations Manager of a staffing service. I was getting job orders and placing qualified applicants. I even helped with her mentoring program and taught the training classes sometimes.) Needless to say, this was very stressful for me, which probably contributed to me being tired all the time.

As a result, I began looking for employment elsewhere. I landed a position at McLeod Regional Medical Center in the pharmacy department as a secretary. I was so excited, because this was an excellent place to work during this time. I began my new job in Feb of 1993. However, I was lacking in performing some of my job duties. It was the typing. I was making too many mistakes because it was hard for me to see (I did not realize this at the time). The director of the pharmacy department did not want to fire me; instead he found another position for me within the hospital. He said I was a good employee, the fit just wasn't right.

So, in April, I began working in the file room of the radiology department. The job was more physically demanding, but I did not mind. I was trained and I thought I was doing a good job. There were some complaints and I did my best to correct the problem areas. One day I was putting files up and I blacked out in the file room. I did not realize this until one of my co-workers came in and saw me on the floor. The next week as I was taking the shortcut (through the ER) I realized how exhausted I was. I figured it was because I was so busy with getting the kids ready for school and running back and forth taking them to school and daycare on my breaks. However, one day, a nurse in the ER asked if I was okay as I was walking through. I responded that I was just a little tired, but fine. She came around her desk and grabbed me and took me into a room. She took my temperature and it was 103.5. She informed me that I could not work like that and that I should go over to Employee Health for treatment. I informed my supervisor and did as I was instructed. They took my temp again, and said I had a cold and to go home, drink plenty of liquids and get some rest. I did as I was told. The next morning, I got up and did the same thing (I got the girls ready and dropped them off at school, then went to work. I was not in a position to miss work since I was still in the probation period).

As I was walking through the ER the nurse stopped me and asked if I went to Employee Health. I responded that I had and told her what they told me. She took my temp again and it was 103 so she sent me back to Employee Health. She said she would call them to notify them that I would be coming and that they should not send me home without treatment. I went over and they checked me out and said I had a sinus infection. I went home with a prescription and was told to take Tylenol for the fever. I followed the advice and returned to work the next morning.

This time when I walked through the ER, the nurse grabbed me and took me to a room for the third time. She asked me if I realized that I was wobbling when I walked. She said they have been watching me and I was stumbling when I walked. I told her that I was just tired. She had me put a gown on and said she would inform my supervisor why I was not at work. About 30-45 minutes later my supervisor came in to talk with me. A while later a doctor came in and examined me. She asked me to get up because she wanted to see me walk. We went into the hallway and she asked me to hold my arms in front of me and walk toward her. Then she asked a question I had not thought about. She said, "Is your gait always this unsteady?" I thought about it for a minute and I told her "no" that it had started about a month before, but I was just tired and needed some rest.

She said she was concerned and that she wanted me to go over to the doctor's office (where the residents treated patients). She told me she would tell them about me and she wanted to make sure I got the correct treatment. I asked her name, Dr. Renee' Watson, so that I could request her as my family doctor. Again, I did as I was told. The doctor who saw me, said I had pharyngitis, ostitis, and laryngitis (throat infection, ear infection and loss of voice). He gave me a prescription for antibiotics and told me not to return to work until the end of the week (this was

Tuesday). I took the medications, but they did not seem to be working, I did not feel better. So I called him and he said he would write a work excuse for a few more days (I was concerned about this since I was still in my 90-day probation period). When I did return to work the next week (It was not my weekend to work), the nurses in the ER stopped me again. This time I went to see Doctor Watson. She examined me and concluded that I had a case of the "old fashioned flu". She said it would probably take four to six weeks for it to run its course and during that time she wanted me at home resting. She would let me return to work on a part time basis if I was better the next time she saw me. I was so upset because I knew my job was in jeopardy. But I did as I was told. I stayed home and rested for six weeks.

During that month and a half something happened. One day my husband had gone to work and the kids were at school so I was alone. I was exhausted all the time and it was hard for me to get out of bed for anything. I had been having some funny feelings in my legs. They felt like they were being stuck with pins and needles. I tried to go to the bathroom one day, and fell flat on my face. I managed to put my tingling legs over the side of the bed using my hands to lift and maneuver them. I finally got my feet on the floor and stood up. I was shocked when my face felt the carpet on the floor. I hit my chin so hard I almost bit through my bottom lip. The first thing I thought about was vacuuming the floor, especially under the bed (This vantage point was enlightening, to say the least). It was horrible. Then it hit me, that I did not stand up and that I had fallen. So, I tried to stand up again. I couldn't get my legs to move. I kept telling them to draw up to my knees so I could pivot and push myself up, but they weren't listening. I had a cordless phone in the room, so I managed to maneuver myself to get the phone (thankfully it was right next to the bed on a night table, right where I had fallen). I called my husband and told him that I was going to call the doctor because the tingling was worse and that I was having trouble moving my legs. I told him not to worry that I was fine and that I would see him when he got off at the normal time. An hour later, to my surprise my husband was walking through the door.

I was propped up in the bed looking at TV and trying to figure out how I was going to get to the kitchen to cook dinner. He looked at me with the saddest eyes I've ever seen. He asked how I was doing and exactly what happened. I told him then he made a phone call. He helped me get dressed and we went to the doctor (he did not go back to work for the day. When I asked him about this, he told me that my health was more important). It took him about two and half hours to get me dressed and into the car. The doctor who saw me was not doctor Watson and he had no idea what was going on. The next week I was scheduled to see Doctor Watson (which made me feel so much better). When she looked at the notes, she told me that she had an idea of what the problem may be. She advised that I would need to get an MRI to be sure. So we made an appointment to see a neurologist as soon as possible (but the soonest appointment we could get was almost two months away).

During my absence from work, I kept in touch with my supervisor and made sure she was informed of what was happening with me. Meanwhile, I was only on the schedule part time per my doctor's excuse. I returned to work on a Monday morning, since we (the supervisor and I) had decided it would be best for me to work the morning rather than afternoon shift. At the end of my shift, the director of the Radiology department called me and my immediate supervisor into his office. I was terminated for willfully not performing my job duties. I expected them to fire me since I had missed time due to being sick while I was still on probation (However, they could have just told me not to return, instead of having me go through all the effort it took to go to work and perform my job).

I left McLeod and went to the employment office to file a claim. I was angry. I felt I was treated unfairly and had not been given a chance to prove myself. The fact that I worked in a hospital meant that I could have gotten sick from being around patients, but obviously that was not taken into consideration. The matter-of-fact manner in which I was terminated really hurt. Especially in light of the fact that I was coming to work tired and doing the very best I could. They had complimented me on my professionalism dealing with the doctors and patients and how quickly I learned the system, but in the end, none of that mattered.

As if not having a job wasn't a big enough problem, I learned that I would be penalized for eight weeks and would not be receiving a check. This meant half our family's income was suddenly gone. I am glad we did not have an excessive amount of bills. However, I appealed the decision and the representatives of McLeod and I had a hearing. To my surprise the Director of Radiology came and he informed the administrator that I was given every opportunity to do my job, but I refused which led to my termination. I told my side of things and explained that I got sick and was ordered out of work by my physician. I also informed them of the pending MRI test and results. The outcome was not in my favor. This was hard to deal with.

In the duration, I went to the appointment with the neurologist. My mother took me to the doctor since my husband was at work and I was no allowed to drive. The tingling in my legs was not as intense by this time, but movement was still difficult. When we arrived at his office, I was so tired. It took me thirty minutes to walk about 30 feet (from the front door to the window to sign in and get things started so I could be seen.). I was using a walker and physically moving my legs by dragging or pulling my pants leg with my hands to move forward. It was a slow go of things and took a lot of energy.

Once I was in the back with the doctor he looked at my symptoms and did a neurological exam. He then performed a nerve-conduction study. He also scheduled MRI's for the upper and lower spine with and without contrast. I went to McLeod and got the tests done then came back to see the doctor within 3 weeks. My mother and I had discussed what we thought could be wrong. I had a few medical books at home and everything I read pointed to MS. My mother was concerned how I would raise my children if it was indeed MS (she did not have any faith in my spouse). However, we would not receive a diagnosis of MS, that day. In fact, the doctor told us that I was having a classic stress-conversion reaction. Imagine the surprise of my mother and I? We asked questions and he informed me that I had a stressful life and that could account for the problems I was having. Naturally, I wanted to know if he thought I was crazy or if he thought it was all in my mind. He explained that he did not think that at all and that he encouraged us to get a second opinion.

When I saw Dr. Watson and she saw his report, she asked what I wanted to do. I eagerly informed her that I wanted a second opinion. She explained that she had another neurologist in mind. I agreed to see him and then we started talking about how I would make necessary changes in my life. She encouraged me to file for disability, since it was obvious, that it would be a while before I could work given my current state. She asked how the children were being cared for. I explained that my husband's Aunt was cooking and bringing food to us on a daily basis (thank goodness for Aunt Illa and Uncle Andy). The girls were old enough to understand that I was sick and tried to make it easier for me. My husband, Carl, did everything else. During the day when I was home alone, I did as much as I could, but it took a long time to sort and wash a load of laundry. I was unable to get them out of the dryer, so I left them until my husband came home and I would have him bring the clothes to me and I would fold them.

Ironically, even though my mother and I were not on the best of terms, she allowed my baby sister to come to my house on the weekends to help me get things done (Tami made life so much easier for me during this time). My doctor had suggested this and it was good for me and my family. It gave me a chance to spend time with my sister and my girls just adored having her around. They would plan things during the week that they wanted to do on the weekend. However, others thought I was faking and trying to get attention. They did not understand that I was not in full control of my body. One day I could walk and they next I might not be able to.

I cheered up once I meet Dr. Demichele. He was a small man with salt and peppered hair who wore jeans and tennis shoes to work. He looked at my MRI results from the other neurologist and ordered an MRI of the C-spine. He gave me orders for a host of other tests including Lyme disease and other stuff that I had never heard of. I went home full of questions. So I delved into my medical books. I saw him in 3 weeks to get the test results. I was not surprised when he said, "You have one of two things, either MS or a brain tumor." Then he showed me the film. He explained that he wanted a better look so I was scheduled for another MRI of the C-spine with contrast.

I left the office in a daze. Based on everything I had read, I was praying for the brain tumor. My thinking was, as long as it was not malignant, they would shave my head, remove it, and I would be fine and could get my life back. I knew that MS was unpredictable and meant a life of uncertainty, which was something I did not want. There was too much going on in our lives for this to be happening.

My husband worked a full time job to pay the bills, but his chosen career was a musician/songwriter. He was doing shows out of town with his group and they were under contract. It was all so promising and it looked like things were finally about to take off musically. He and I discussed our lives and any medical consequences. He had been raised in New York and his mother had musical contacts there. She had been encouraging him to move away from Florence for the sake of his music career. I agreed that we should move, but I wanted to move to Atlanta, while she suggested New York. I felt New York was too big and too expensive. Not to mention, I did not really want to raise my children in New York, but I was willing to make the move for him.

Anyway, when I saw Dr. DeMichele, he confirmed my worst fear. I had Multiple Sclerosis, relapsing and remitting, as it was called then. November 1993 was a hard month. The following week I met with Social Security and completed my application for disability. It was sobering for the family (immediate) to finally know what the problem was. We, my husband and I, explained to the children how difficult it might be for me to do things sometimes. We didn't expect them to understand everything, since they were only six and four.

In January 1994, I was admitted to the hospital because I could not walk, could barely see and was too fatigued to do anything. Unfortunately, Dr.Demichele was out of town. His partner saw me and he declared that I had chronic progressive MS and would be wheelchair bound in three years and nursing home bound in five years. This was completely different from what Dr. Demichele had told me and I was angry. He had given me a death sentence and said as much. This was the first hospitalization for the MS and I decided to prove him wrong. My husband got a job transfer to New Jersey and we were going to move to further his music career. Since I fell and hit my head on a regular basis, I was not allowed to be alone for long periods. As a result, when my husband took the transfer, the girls and I moved in with my grandmother. The girls really missed their father and sometimes it was very difficult to deal with. But, he called everyday to make sure he spoke to us. He was gone for a total of 7 months and we saw him four times. He would surprise us and make the twelve-hour drive to

Florence, SC. The girls and I were always so happy to see him. It was stressful and difficult to coordinate the move to New Jersey. There were financial and health considerations which could not be worked out. As a result, my husband moved back to SC.

Dr. D (DeMichele) was concerned about my quality of life. As a result, he prescribed Beteseron. I tried the medication, but after a while, realized I was not tolerating it well. We decided I would manage the disease with steroids for the time being. So, once a month, I went to the doctor to get my steroids. How was I doing? I had flare ups on a regular basis. I was in and out of the hospital. I had good and bad days and I gained a lot of weight, but at least I would walk with the help of assistive devices. I had been approved for Social Security disability after a couple of appeals and this took a weight off of my shoulders.

We finally bought a house the following year. I was bored being at home. I had started doing little things to keep busy. I began looking for part time work, but no one would hire me after speaking with one of my past employers. It infuriated me that I was getting a bad reference saying that I could not work because of my illness. All I really needed was the chance. After a while, a staffing service gave me an opportunity. I got a two-week assignment which turned into a permanent part time position. Ironically,

I worked as the office assistant for a doctor who did disability determination medical exams. It was interesting to see the process. I learned about different conditions and how to do neurological examinations.

My employer was aware of my medical condition and allowed me to work around this. Unfortunately, I passed out at work one day and was taken to the hospital. I was admitted and released after a week to be on homebound for three months. I had a nurse, and two therapists come to the house on a daily basis. It turns out I had a major problem with my hypoglycemia. It took a while to recover from this.

I began to volunteer at the girl's school. It was so fulfilling. I went one day a week. It was a joy to be able to do it and the children understood that I had trouble walking and that was why I used a walker or cane. By the time, my oldest daughter was in the sixth grade, even the parents thought I was employed at the school. The students knew who I was. I was asked to chaperone the sixth grade trip. Unfortunately, I got sick while on the out-of-town trip, but the children helped take care of me. It was amazing and it made me cry. I didn't realize how much they cared.

In 2001, we decided to move to Atlanta, Ga. The students at the school were so sad. They asked if they could move with us. Unfortunately, because of some work related injuries, my husband had difficulty finding work in Florence. He left on a Tuesday evening and began working on a Thursday in Atlanta. That turned into a permanent position. The move was good for us, unlike the move to New Jersey, which never happened. Naturally, the kids didn't feel the same way. They were upset about leaving their friends. In 2004, I found out about the Shepherd MS Institute, thanks to a co-worker. I have been a patient every since. Currently, I am taking Tysarbi, after trying Betaseron, Avonex and Copaxone, to help manage my MS. I was having a problem with a spastic left arm, but that has since resolved. I am having issues with the vision in my left eye.

2001 to Present Day

In April of 2001, my family was in an automobile accident, which resulted in a left knee injury for me. Needless to say, I was not a happy camper. I was fine and could move all of my extremities, before the accident. Then, we got hit and were spun around 180 degrees. After that nothing moved. Since we got hit on my side of the car, my door was stuck and the firefighters had to pop it open. Once that was done and they helped me to my legs, then the big surprise came. I leaned against the frame of the car to steady myself as I prepared myself to step up onto the curb. But that never happened. Instead, I quickly fell to my knees and hit the curb. Boy did that hurt! So I was taken to the hospital. I was disappointed with the level of service received in the ER for a MS flare.

I explained that I lived with MS and the looks on the faces of the medical staff was scary to me. At one point they fully admitted that they did not know how to treat me. So, I explained what to do. I said, "…give me a gram of steroids, watch me for a while and let me go home (since I did not want to be hospitalized so far away from my family, as it was a logistical nightmare)." Yes, I know that is not the treatment. But, it must have sounded right to them, because they did it. I was happy to get home. I spent the next couple of weeks recovering slowly. I slowly regained movement of my legs and I continued to do the physical therapy exercises I had learned when I got my initial diagnosis.

But, I managed to find part time work (just two days a week and when the other staff was on vacation). The only negative thing with this employment was that there was a flight of stairs, which required climbing at times. Since I had been honest and informed my employer of my Multiple Sclerosis, he was sympathetic to my needs (which is sometimes not the case). Climbing the stairs and other walking in the office aggravated my knee injury. After seeing an orthopedist for several months and concluding that nothing else could be done, we came up with a solution. The treatment was surgery, something I did not want. But eventually, walking with a limp, not being able to sit, stand, lye down or even sleep without pain, won over my desire for the operation. As a result of that car accident, I suffered a severely torn ligament on the left side of my left knee. So, in January of 2002, I had the surgery after all other treatments had failed. After months of physical therapy, I felt so much better. I was back to walking for exercise and not using my cane anymore. I even landed a new job after I fully recovered. I worked for a dental group (a few days a week at the corporate office). This allowed me to have a measure of independence and feel like a productive member of society.

Unfortunately, in August of 2005, I was involved in another automobile accident (yes, cars aim for me so I rarely drive). The same knee was injured. Imagine my orthopedic doctor's surprise when I came back to him with the same knee injured. The injury was a little different. But, since I did the outpatient physical therapy and took the medications, with no relief, surgery was the last resort. (When I say, I would rather have a baby than have knee surgery, I am not joking). So, on July 19, 2006 we did the outpatient surgery. But, on July 20, my father was put into a medication induced coma after a stroke in South Carolina. What did I do? The wrong thing. I sat in the backseat of the car with my leg propped against the headrest of the front passenger seat for the four-hour trip. (I would not risk not having a chance to say goodbye to my father). Do I regret the decision to go? No. But, I know that from a medical point of view, it was the wrong thing to do and I would discourage another person from doing anything like that.

We came back to Atlanta on Sunday evening (July 22, 2006). I went to see my doctor for my post-op appointment on Monday morning July 23, 2006. When I told him about my weekend, he was visibly upset with me. However, he said at least I used the leg and that is a good thing. But, he fussed at me, as I expected. All I could do was take it, since I knew I was wrong (cookies would not fix this).

However, the good thing about all of this is that I was seeing doctor Thrower at the Shepherd Center's MS Institute.

UPDATE: As of the printing of this book, I am back on Tysabri. I stopped taking it for a few years. During the early stages of administering Tysabri it was a big deal od someone converted to positive for the JC virus. I did just that. So my family and I though I had a short time to live. As a result, I stopped the Tysabri and tried the oral medications (Aubagio and Tecfidera). My doctor decided that Gilenya was not right for me.

Unfortunately, I am allergic to all of them! So it is a needle and Tysabri for me. Thankfully, they have fine-tuned the screening process for PML and even though I'm positive for the JC virus, I'm not in danger of getting PML. My risk is low. So, I head to Shepherd once a month to get my infusion. It is getting increasingly hard to find a vein, but we do what we can so I can get my medicine.

I worry that I will run out of options since I have so many allergies. I usually don't think about it too much until they have to find a vein (that is a task). But I'm happy to be able to get something to help slow the progression of the disease. I try to stay positive and optimistic at all times, even though my life is an uncertainty in some aspects.

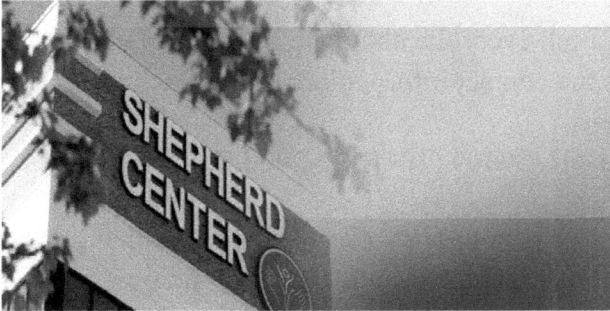

(copyright-Shepherd Center brochure-shepherd.org)

I began going to the Shepherd Center because a co-worker, Crystal Powell, noticed the way I walked one day (This was when I worked for a dental group). She watched for a while (she told me) before she approached me. She asked me if I had a neurological problem. I explained that I have vertigo (because of where my MS plaques are located). She informed me that she had a son living with her who has MS. Then she asked who my doctor was. I explained that I had not found one (that I liked as much as Dr. DeMichele) that I could work with, yet. She immediately suggested that I try the Shepherd Center and gave me Dr. Thrower's name. Naturally, I went home to research the center and find out all I could. I called and made an appointment. This was in 2004 and I have been going ever since. I have participated in several research studies because I feel this is how I can give back. In addition, I volunteer with the National MS Society when time allows.

I tell everyone about the Shepherd Center. Here is the contact information: 2020 Peachtree Road Northeast
Atlanta, GA 30309 (404) 352-2020

It is a private, not-for-profit hospital specializing in medical treatment, research and rehabilitation for people with spinal cord and brain injury, multiple sclerosis, spine and chronic pain and other neuromuscular conditions (shepherd.org) which was founded in 1975. It is located right next door to Piedmont hospital and is ranked by U.S. News and World Report among the top 10 rehabilitation hospitals in the nation. While care by the staff and faculty of the MS institute is great, there are other benefits to going to the Shepherd Center. For instance, there is a gym, which is available for use.

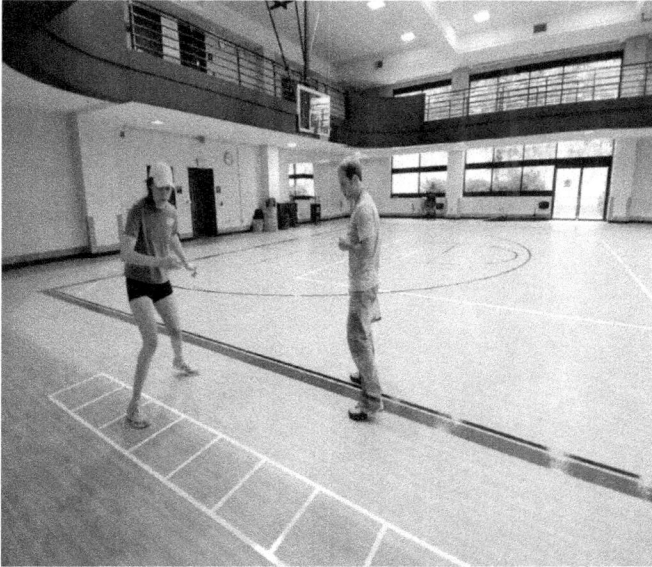

Livingston Gym. Photo courtesy of Shepherd Center

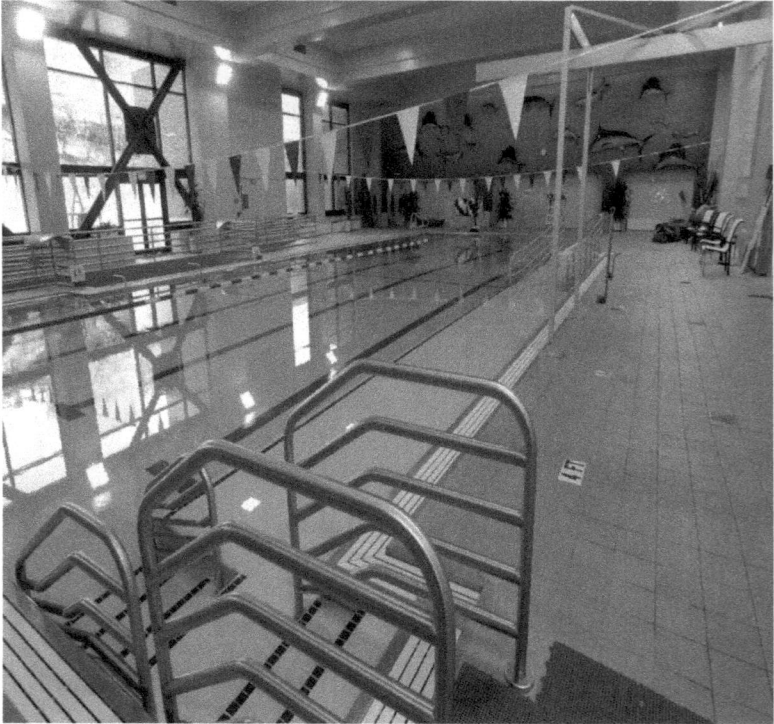

Shepherd Center pool. Photo courtesy of Shepherd Center

There is also a pool for aquatic aerobics.

From July 2006 to January 2018 I have had numerous MS flare ups. I've had some serious medical incidents not related to my MS and I've come though them. My MS baseline is no longer where it used to be. I've moved into a different type of MS. I'm going on 25 years living with this disease.

However, I began experiencing something that had me worried about my heart. I felt pain in my chest. So, after seeing a cardiologist and determining that my heart was a diagnosis was made. The doctor said I have a "MS hug".

"A what?" I asked.

She said that it often can feel like heart symptoms, but she explained what was happening. She said there are small muscles between the ribs and when a person has muscles spasms here, then you feel pain and tightening pressure. She mentioned that because of where the pain occurs that it often mimics a heart attack. She commended me for seeing a cardiologist and ruling out any heart issue. The fact that is was coming and going for days was an indicator that it was not a heart issue. I was so shocked since my pain was crippling. It was so hard to breathe.

We talked about triggers (stress, overwork or being very tired) and what I needed to avoid. Then she briefly went over some things to try (drinking plenty of water, getting rest, deep breathing exercises, comfortable clothing). When he discussed how long I had been dealing with it, she prescribed something for pain. I took it that night and wow, for the first time on months, I could take a deep breathe without pain. It felt so good.

Interviews of Persons living with MS

My answers (as if you haven't read enough about me)

What was your occupation before MS was diagnosed?
Office worker

How long have you been living with MS?
Almost 20 years. But we can actually trace the symptoms back to when I was a child.

What are your physical limitations?
I am currently ambulatory with the assistance of a quad-cane.

What are your other medical issues (hypertensions and so forth)?
Hmm… let's see. I'll just list the major ones, which include hypertension, asthma, severe allergies, migraines, sciatica and angina (I think that is enough).

What were the first symptoms you experienced?
I did not realize it, but the problems started with the vision in my left eye. To this day, I have major vision disturbances from blindness to mildly blurry.

How long did it take for you to get diagnosed?
About 6 months

Are you currently taking any medication to manage the MS?
Tysabri infusions every 4 weeks.

How often do you have flare ups?
Since the criteria for a flare up involves symptoms that last for more than 24 hours, at least 2-3 per month. Generally speaking, these are not severe and I can manage with rest and doing my physical therapy exercises. However, sometimes (rarely) they are large enough to put me down for a week or more. In these cases, I go to the hospital for treatment.

Did you immediately begin taking medication once you received the MS diagnosis?
Yes, I started out with Beteseron, which was a new drug at the time.

What is most affected by the MS for you?
I have spasticity on my left side and my memory. I also have a major problem with my balance and weakness in my legs, which affects my gait.

What kind of support do you have?
My immediate family is always there for me. I have other family members, congregation members and the support of outpatient medical staff and friends. I am very fortunate.

Do you have a caregiver?
Yes, I live with my husband who helps with my daily needs and puts up with me (poor man).

How many times have you been hospitalized for the MS?
I have lost track of the hospitalizations for MS.

Have you been able to keep working or have concessions been made for you?
I used to work with a company which hires disabled Americans. J. Lodge was been a blessing. I could work from home and they understand my situation. I plan on staying with them until I am no longer able to work. However, I had to resign for other reasons.

UPDATE: At the printing of this book, I am no longer working with a company. I am a freelance graphic designer and editor.

How would you describe living with MS?
I believe we are all given challenges in life. But, MS, has given me a level of determination that is unmatched by anything else. I am often fussed at for being too independent. But, I refuse to be a burden to others (At least not intentionally). As a result, I have a fiercely independent spirit (which is not always good, even though admirable to some). I will say that MS has made me determined to do the things that I love and want to do. It has also taught me not to procrastinate, since I never know what tomorrow will be like. My life is not without challenges, but overall, I'm happy because it could be so much worse.

But, since MS is such an unpredictable disease, I am going to relate some other stories.

The Experiences of Others

Alicia-Atlanta, Ga
(As told by the patient)

In Feb. 1990, I broke a vegan diet because I changed jobs working 3rd shift. I stopped by McDonald's and picked up junk food and a diet coke. My left torso began to become numb and my vision started going bad. My doctor said that I started having signs of MS. I then read about aspartame, then quit because the info said that I could get MS and depression. I had signs of both. I had a child in 1995, and lost the ability to walk well. I had an MRI in 2008 and my neurologist confirmed that I have MS. It has gotten worse over the years. As with other MS patients, I can't stand heat. I purchased a book by Judy Graham that told me about vitamins I needed to take. Evening Primrose Oil and Vitamin E is a must daily or my balance isn't good. Also I had to cut out a lot of fried food, milk products, and sugar. If I fall, it is because my balance is off. I stumble a lot. Once I broke my wrist. But, I must always keep the Primrose and Vitamin E or I have a really hard time balancing myself. I am always tired and lack motivation. My arms look very bad. After breaking my wrist, I at times try to cook and I tend to burn myself. I can have a full night's sleep but I am always yawning. I need my cane when I walk away from my van. When I go shopping, my husband or my son always gives me the shopping cart so that I can get in the store.

In 2008, as I was leaving my house, I fell out of the door and landed on my hand. My husband had to leave work to take me to the emergency room. The doctor said that I suffered a clean break on my wrist. In 2009, I went to pay the gas bill. As I was leaving, I noticed the hand rails didn't go to the last stair. I attempted to walk down and fell on my face. The security guard ran out and helped me. She asked me if I wanted an ambulance, but I felt that I didn't need it. I spoke with my sister who is an RN and she told me that I needed to go to the hospital in case an infection sets in. I had my husband take me and it wasn't infected.

John-South Carolina

John resides in Florence South Carolina in a nursing home. He has chronic progressive MS. His personality is always upbeat in spite of his medical condition and he is always helpful. When I called him about doing this interview, he readily agreed to do it. Even though he could not hold the phone himself, he took the time and energy to answer my questions. I remember meeting him as a young teen. I even remember when he got sick and the problems he began having. Since we were in the same congregation, we saw each other on a regular basis. He was in a wheelchair and I was on a walker. It always made me happy to see him because he is so positive and full of life.

His interview follows:

What was your occupation before MS was diagnosed?
Mechanic

How long have you been living with MS?
More than 20 years

What are your physical limitations?
Wheelchair bound

What are you other medical issues (hypertensions and so forth)?
N/A

What were the first symptoms you experienced?
Pains in wrist, hands and feet, blind in one eye, right

How long did it take for you to get diagnosed?
2-3 years

Are you currently taking any medication to manage the MS?
Acne medicine

How often do you have flare ups?
1 per year

Did you immediately begin taking medication once you received the MS diagnosis?
Went to Germany for bee pollen treatments, took Betaseron and Copaxone

What is most affected by the MS for you?
Self feeding, spasticity and fatigue

What kind of support do you have?
Nursing home staff, friends in congregation and my wife.

Do you have a caregiver?
6 years in a nursing home

How many times have you been hospitalized for the MS?
8-9 times

Have you been able to keep working or have concessions been made for you?
No longer able to work.

How would you describe living with MS?
Rough, robs you of the things you want to do.

UPDATE: As of the printing of this book, sadly John passed away in 2017. He was a fighter and I miss him.

Caregiver Interviews

Carl-My Spouse

How long have you been helping to care for an MS patient?

I've been caring for the patient for almost 25 years.

Do you find the MS patient to be difficult? If so, in what way?

It's not so much as the patient being difficult but more so that the patient fights so hard for independence that they don't see when they are putting themselves in harms way.

What is your greatest fear for the patient?

My greatest fear is that she may injure herself trying to do too much at a time.

Can you tell when the patient has done too much and will pay for it later?

Most of the time I can tell when she has done too much and it will cost her later. Sometimes I will let her do it without saying anything because I know that what she's doing means a lot to her.

Do you know the signs of a flare up?

Most of the time there are small tell tale signs of a flare up, but are not seen often.

What do you want for the MS patient?

I'd like the patient to take it easy more. I'd like her to work on her diet and cut down more on her consumption of meats (outside of fish), or maybe eliminate it from her diet. At least for a year. Although doctors have no clue to what causes MS, I have a strong gut feeling that less consumption of meat will give her stronger days where she is more in control. I would be willing to adhere to the same diet to give support.

Jasmine –My Youngest Daughter

How long have you been helping to care for an MS patient? It's been about 24 years. I really started when I was about 8 yrs old.

Do you find the MS patient to be difficult? If so, in what way? Sometimes, yes. We try to tell her of things we don't think she should be doing, but she's such a fighter that she tries to do it anyway. Sometimes she proves us wrong and she can do whatever it is, and sometimes she has consequences where she'll fall out or overdo it and have a small exacerbation.

What is your greatest fear for the patient? That one day she will think that she can do a task, but not realize how weak she is and really hurt herself. I got a small glimpse of that when she broke her ankle a few years ago.

Can you tell when the patient has done too much and will pay for it later? Usually yes. She becomes even more fatigued and she becomes more unbalanced.

Do you know the signs of a flare up? Yes. She may drop things more or her knees will buckle a lot. If she loses the feeling in her arm, she unconsciously holds it a certain way across her torso. There have been many times where I have to ask if she has lost feeling before she realizes it. Also, if she stays in the bed too late in the morning, I can tell that she's not having a good day as well.

What do you want for the MS patient? I want for her to be able to live normally, but I understand that it is a progressive illness. I just want for her to be able to function to the best of her ability on her own, but not be afraid to ask for help if she needs it. We understand that sometimes she will have difficulty and we'll always be here to help.

Marilyn —My oldest daughter

How long have you been helping to care for an MS patient?

For 24 years I've been helping to take care of my mom.

Do you find the MS patient to be difficult? If so, in what way?

My mom can be difficult a lot of the time, but mostly because she likes to try to do things her particular way, and sometimes she doesn't realize that she would do too much and tire herself out. It's hard for her to accept help and realize that we want her to perform her best and sometimes, that means taking it easy and doing less activity.

What is your greatest fear for the patient?

I get worried that one day she won't be able to get around at all. Her mobility has diminished slowly over the last several years and I know that she worries about a time when she will barely be able to do anything at all. With a young grandson, I know that is something that she worries about too.

Can you tell when the patient has done too much and will pay for it later?

I can definitely tell. She starts to wobble a lot when she walks, or can't walk a straight line and has to stop and collect herself. Sometimes she'll start gasping for air as well when her allergies and asthma are getting to her. When her knees hurt, she rubs them subconsciously.

Do you know the signs of a flare up?
It seems like when she has a lot of tingling in one of her limbs, a flare up is coming. Also, she tends to sleep a lot more just before a flare up.

What do you want for the MS patient?
I'd really just like for my mom to be able to live a normal life, but I know that in the world that we live in now, it's impossible. I'd like for her to be able to enjoy her day to day life. I'd like for her to be able to take my son to the park and run and play with him, but for now I'll take her being able to mentally and emotionally handle the changes that are going on right now in the best way. She has a very strong spiritual background and I know that that helps her to keep a positive attitude in her day to day life and I just want to be able to support her and continue to be a source of encouragement to her. I want her to know that she isn't alone in her struggle and I'm always there to help, even when she doesn't want it.

Medical Stuff

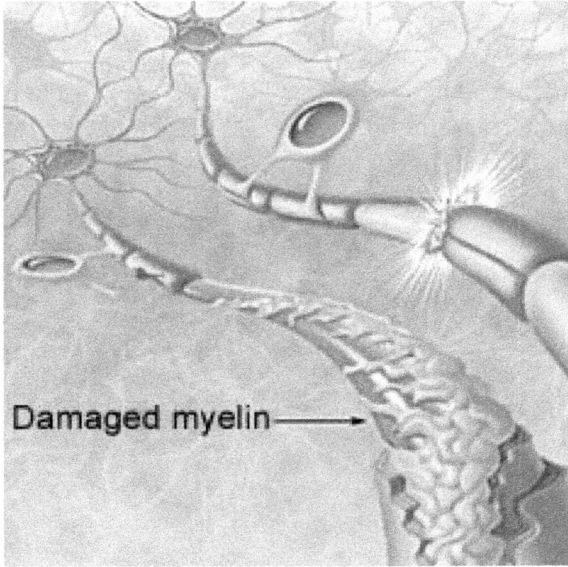

Damaged myelin——→

Films

The symptoms of MS vary greatly from person to person, depending on where the damaged nerve fibers are located.

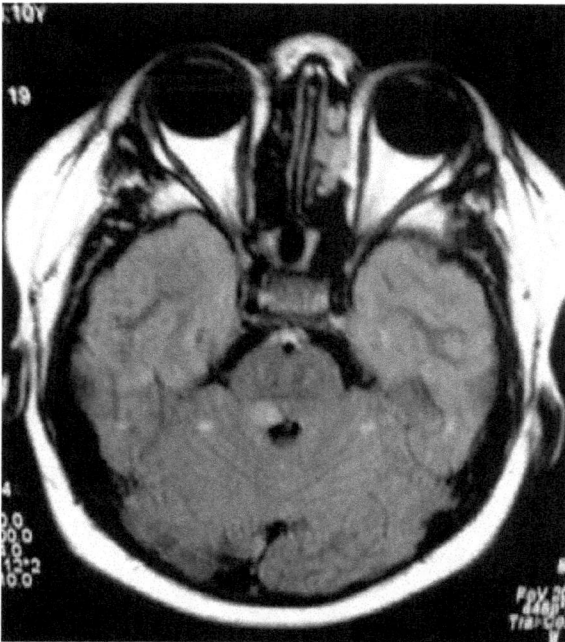

lesions involving the cerebellum and brain stem courtesy of WebMD.

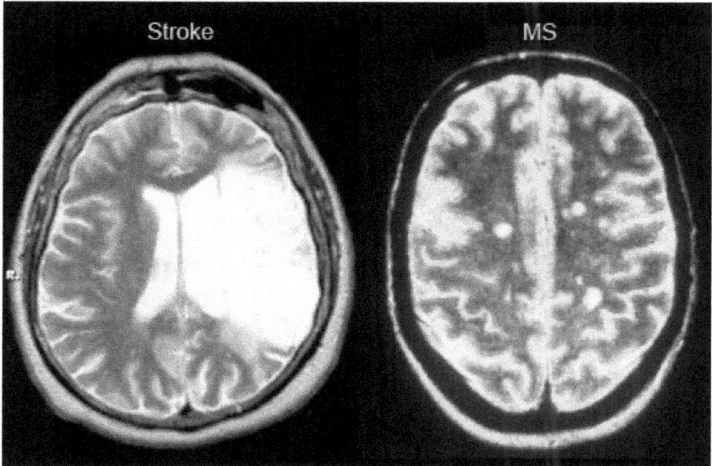

Courtesy of WebMD-difference between a stroke and
MS plaques.

Symptoms

Here is a list of general symptoms:

- Tingling
- Numbness
- Loss of balance
- Weakness in one or more limbs
- Blurred or double vision
- Slurred speech
- Sudden onset of paralysis
- Lack of coordination
- Cognitive difficulties

As the disease progresses, other symptoms may include fatigue, muscle spasms, sensitivity to heat, sexual dysfunction and changes in thinking or perception.

- **Fatigue**. This is a characteristic and common symptom of MS. It is typically present in the midafternoon and may consist of increased muscle weakness, mental fatigue, sleepiness, or drowsiness. Physical exhaustion is not related to the amount of work performed; and many patients with MS complain of extreme fatigue even after a good night's sleep.

• **Heat sensitivity** . Heat sensitivity (the appearance or worsening of symptoms when exposed to heat, like a hot shower) occurs in most people with MS.

• **Spasticity** . Muscle spasms are a common and often debilitating symptom of MS. Spasticity usually affects the muscles of the legs and arms, and may interfere with a persons ability to move those muscles freely.

• **Dizziness**. Many people with MS complain of feeling "off balance" or lightheaded. Occasionally they may experience the feeling that they or their surroundings are spinning; this is called vertigo. These symptoms are caused by damage in the complex nerve pathways that coordinate vision and other inputs into the brain that are needed to maintain balance.

• **Impaired thinking**. Problems with thinking occur in about half of people with MS. For most, this means slowed thinking, decreased concentration, or decreased memory. Approximately 10% of people with the disease have severe impairment that significantly impairs their ability to carry out tasks of daily living.

• **Vision problems**. Vision problems are relatively common in people with MS. In fact, one vision problem, optic neuritis, occurs in 55% of people with the condition. This can result in blurring or graying of vision or blindness in one eye. However, most vision problems in MS do not lead to blindness.

- **Abnormal sensations**. Many people with MS experience abnormal sensations such as "pins and needles," numbness, itching, burning, stabbing, or tearing pains. Fortunately, most of these symptoms, while aggravating, are not life-threatening or debilitating and can be managed or treated.

- **Speech and swallowing problems** . People with MS often have swallowing difficulties. In many cases, they are associated with speech problems as well. They are caused by damaged nerves that normally aid in performing these tasks.

- **Tremors**. Fairly common in people with MS, tremors can be debilitating and difficult to treat.

- **Difficulty walking**. Gait disturbances are amongst the most common symptoms of MS. Mostly this problem is related to muscle weakness and/or spasticity, but having balance problems or numbness in your feet can also make walking difficult.

Other rare symptoms include breathing problems and seizures (WebMD, 2010)

Multiple Sclerosis: Recognizing Multiple Sclerosis

What Are the Types of Symptoms?
It is helpful to divide the symptoms into three categories: primary, secondary, and tertiary.

Primary symptoms are a direct result of the demyelination process. This impairs the transmission of electrical signals to muscles (to allow them to move appropriately) and the organs of the body (allowing them to perform normal functions.) The symptoms include: weakness, tremors, tingling, numbness, loss of balance, vision impairment, paralysis, and bladder or bowel problems. Medication, rehabilitation, and other treatments can help keep many of these symptoms under control.

Secondary symptoms result from primary symptoms. For example, paralysis (a primary symptom) can lead to bedsores (pressure sores) and bladder or urinary incontinence problems can cause frequent, recurring urinary tract infections. These symptoms can be treated, but the ideal goal is to avoid them by treating the primary symptoms.

Tertiary symptoms are the social, psychological, and vocational complications associated with the primary and secondary symptoms. Depression, for example, is a common problem among people with MS.

What Causes the Symptoms?
Demyelination, or deterioration of the protective sheath that surrounds nerve fibers, can occur in any part of the brain or spinal cord. The symptoms that people with MS experience depend on the affected

area. Demyelination in the nerves that send messages to the muscles causes problems with movement (motor symptoms), while demyelination along the nerves that carry sensory messages to the brain causes disturbances in sensation.

Are Symptoms the Same in Every Person?

Multiple sclerosis follows a varied and unpredictable course. In many people, the disease starts with a single symptom, followed by months or even years without any progression of symptoms. In others, the symptoms become worse within weeks or months.

It is important to understand that although a wide range of symptoms can occur, a given individual may experience only some of the symptoms and never have others. Some symptoms may occur once, resolve, and never return. Because MS is such an individual disease, it is not helpful to compare yourself with other people who have MS.

Symptoms

By Mayo Clinic staff

Signs and symptoms of multiple sclerosis vary widely, depending on the location of affected nerve fibers. Multiple sclerosis signs and symptoms may include:

• Numbness or weakness in one or more limbs, which typically occurs on one side of your body at a time or the bottom half of your body

• Partial or complete loss of vision, usually in one eye at a time, often with pain during eye movement (optic neuritis)

• Double vision or blurring of vision

• Tingling or pain in parts of your body

• Electric-shock sensations that occur with certain head movements

• Tremor, lack of coordination or unsteady gait

• Fatigue

• Dizziness

Most people with multiple sclerosis, particularly in the beginning stages of the disease, experience relapses of symptoms, which are followed by periods of complete or partial remission. Signs and symptoms of multiple sclerosis often are triggered or worsened by an increase in body temperature.

http://www.mayoclinic.com/health/multiple-sclerosis/ds00188/dsection=symptoms

Neurologist Interview

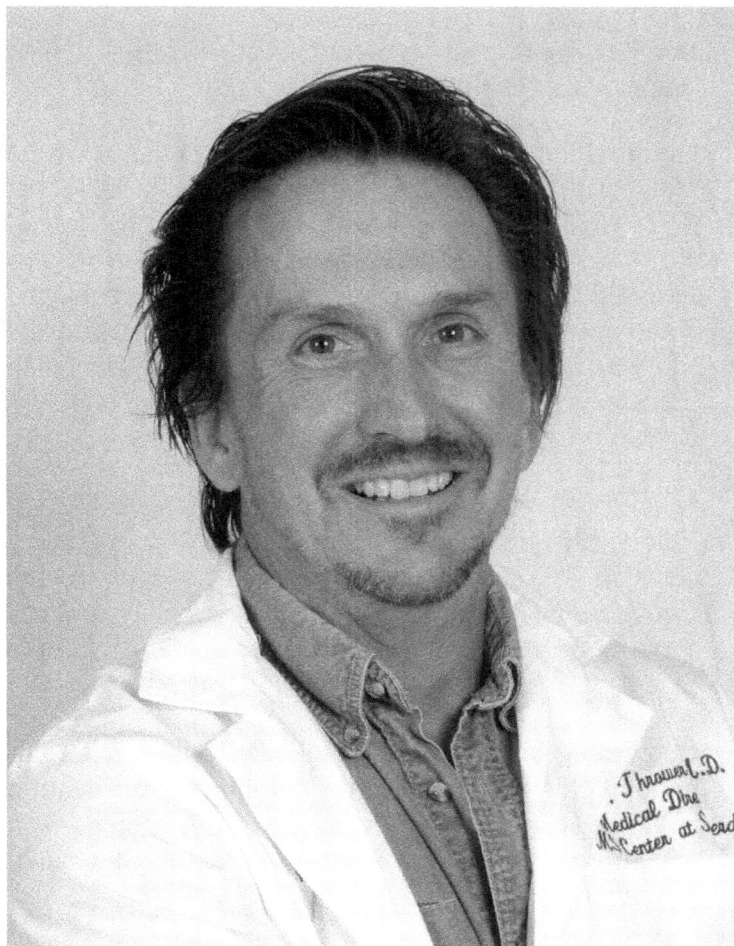

Ben Thrower, M.D., medical director of MS Institute at Shepherd. Photo Courtesy of Shepherd Center

Medical Director
Multiple Sclerosis Institute at Shepherd

**Dr. Thrower is the Medical Director of the
Andrew C. Carlos MS Institute at Shepherd.**

He previously served as the Medical Director of the
Holy Family Multiple Sclerosis Institute in Spokane,
WA. In Spokane he was the Chair of the Inland
Northwest Chapter of the NMSS. In 2000, he was
awarded the Norm Cohn Hope Chest Award by the
National MS Society, recognizing his work with the
MS community. In 2005, he was the first physician
inductee into the Georgia Chapter of the National MS
Society Volunteer Hall of Fame.

Dr. Thrower is a clinical instructor of neurology at
Emory University and participates actively in clinical
research. He serves on the board of directors of the
Georgia Chapter of the National MS Society and has
served on the board for the Consortium of Multiple
Sclerosis Institutes.

Combining his professional interests with his love of
motorcycles he founded the non-profit organization
HAMS, Hogs Against MS. His wife, Karen, is a
pediatrician. They have three children, Stephanie,
Nathan and Sam.

What made you decide to become a Neurologist?
I became interested in Neurology in medical school,
but was really undecided until my third year. The
brain and human nervous system are just fascinating

to me.

Why specialize in Multiple Sclerosis?
After my residency training in Neurology, my wife
owed the Air Force some payback time for her
scholarship to med school. We found ourselves in
Spokane, Washington, where the prevalence of MS is
quite high. As I began working with more people with
MS, I found it to be exciting and challenging. I also
realized that good MS care meant working with a
comprehensive team, including therapists, Urologists,
case managers and many others. In 1999, I made the
decision to focus exclusively on working with the MS
community and have never regretted it.

How important is attitude and outlook on life to an MS patient?

Every person is faced with challenges in their life,
whether it's physical, emotional or financial. How a
person responds to those challenges may make the
difference between being happy versus being bitter
and angry. MS is by its very nature an unpredictable
disease that can be disabling. One of the challenges
that I see for the person with MS is how to deal with
MS proactively but at the same time not let it become
the absolute focus of a person's life. Some people find
that balance easily while others struggle and may
need the help of a counselor, peer, or spiritual
advisor.

In layman's terms how would you explain what happens in an MS flare up?

An exacerbation in MS is also called a flare-up, attack or relapse. This means that the person has new or worsened neurological symptoms like weakness, numbness or visual loss that lasts for more than 24 hours. Some people with MS experience an increase in symptoms when they have an infection like a common cold, the flu or a bladder infection. These are called pseudo-exacerbations. We use the term relapsing-remitting MS to describe the most common form of MS. Remission would seem to mean that the person is free of all symptoms. Unfortunately, this is not the case. Even when their MS is in remission, most people with MS will still deal with things like fatigue, memory issues or other symptoms left over from prior relapses.

What is the standard treatment for an MS flare up?
The standard treatment for an MS relapse would be a form of steroids called Solumedrol (methylprednisolone) given intravenously over three to five days. Sometimes, a tapering dose of prednisone by mouth is given afterwards. There are other options, including high dose oral steroids, plasma exchange and IV immunoglobulin. Imethylprednislone has been shown to potentially speed up recovery from a relapse but does not change the ultimate degree of recovery.

Would alternative medicine/therapy be helpful to MS patients?

Many people with MS are interested in alternative or complementary therapies. Finding good consumer advice can be challenging. Research is showing that low Vitamin D levels are common in MS and that correcting the problem may help slow the MS process. Regular exercise has been shown to improve energy levels and mood in MS. To help further explore this topic, I highly recommend the book Alternative and Therapies and Multiple Sclerosis by Dr. Allen Bowling.

Where do you see MS research heading in the future?
There are many current research projects looking at different aspects of MS. I expect that we will see several oral medications getting FDA approval over the next few years, including one or two in 2010. Other areas of interest include better medications to manage symptoms, more effective and convenient drugs to slow the course of MS and, hopefully, therapies to repair damage in the brain and spinal cord.

In your opinion, what is the greatest danger to MS patients?
To me, the greatest threat to the person with MS is misinformation or the failure to act. Most people with MS work hard to manage their MS and stay informed about what options they have to treat their MS. Sometimes people get bad information form the internet, friends, family or even healthcare providers. Fortunately, there is a wealth of good information out

there as well through groups like the National MS Society, the MS Foundation and the MS Association of America. Denial is dangerous in MS. I do see the occasional patient who just falls off the radar screen and does nothing to deal with their MS.

What services not currently offered should be made available to MS patients?

Ideally, every person with MS would have access to a comprehensive MS Center where a whole team of healthcare providers would be available. Some people cannot access this type of care due to insurance restrictions, transportation issues or lack of knowledge that such care exists.

Delaying MS Progression -- Full-Length Doctor's Interview

In this full-length doctor's interview, Ben Thrower, M.D., explains how a new drug may be able to slow the progression of Multiple Sclerosis
December 15, 2003
Ivanhoe Broadcast News
Ivanhoe Broadcast News Transcript with Ben Thrower, M.D., Neurologist,
The Shepherd Center, Atlanta, Georgia

What's the idea behind your Multiple Sclerosis research?
Dr. Thrower: [The drug NBI-5788 consists of] an altered peptide ligand, and the idea is that rather than trying to suppress the immune system to treat multiple sclerosis, you're trying to actually take advantage of a natural response that our immune system has. The altered peptide ligand looks a little bit like one of the natural components of the covering of nerve fibers in our brain and spinal cord, something called myelin basic protein. The idea is that the altered peptide ligand will look like myelin basic protein, it will interact with immature white blood cells in our immune system, and actually rather than letting them develop into an aggressive or attacking sort of white blood cell, it will send them down the pathway to being a more regulatory, more protective type of white blood cell.

What does that translate into for the patient?

Dr. Thrower: Hopefully, what it will translate into are fewer MS attacks, no progression of disability, and an MRI that looks stable or better over time.

Is it just for patient in advanced stages?
Dr. Thrower: We don't know with any of our new drugs, ultimately, what types of MS they will be used in, but for a study, you have to pick one particular type. The type of MS that this drug is looking at initially will be people with a very aggressive, inflammatory form of MS. More likely than not, they will be people who are relatively newly diagnosed who have a pretty aggressive up-and-down course to their MS, with an MRI that shows some active inflammation.

What were the results from the first trial?
Dr. Thrower: In the initial trials, what we've seen is that the drug appears to be safe and it appears to suppress the inflammatory activity on MRI.

So, this trial will be taking it a step further to look at the safety of the drug in a larger group of people and again, to look for evidence that we're suppressing that active inflammation on MRI.

Talk about the lesions. Was there a reduction of lesions?
Dr. Thrower: Correct. When we look at lesions on MRI, we talk about lesions that are either actively inflamed or what we call a T2 lesion, which is a lesion that may or may not show active inflammation. What we've seen so far with the studies, with altered

peptide ligand, is that it appears that both of those are suppressed over time.

Is NBI-5788 a new drug?
Dr. Thrower: The only application for the altered peptide ligand has been for multiple sclerosis. The idea of using this goes back a few years, but it really is unique to multiple sclerosis.

How is this study different from the other studies looking at NBI-5788?
Dr. Thrower: This is going to be a larger study. It's a multinational trial primarily based in the United States and Canada, but it will be the first multicenter trial, rather than just focusing on one center with a small group of people with MS. This will be at multiple centers with a large number of people with MS, which should give us a better feeling for its safety and effectiveness.

Based on earlier trials, are there any side effects of taking NBI-5788?
Dr. Thrower: We don't worry too much about side effects. One thing that we'll have to be careful about would be any sort of hypersensitivity reactions with the drug. When we're altering the immune system, not really suppressing it but sending it down a pathway, there's a balance in our immune system between these inflammatory types of cells and these more regulatory types of cells. The more regulatory type of white blood cells also carries with them a little bit of potential for allergies. We think these types of white blood cells are the ones that may regulate

whether someone has, say, hay fever and things like that, so they also may carry with them a little bit of risk of skin reactions, hives and side effects like that.

How is it administered?

Dr. Thrower: The altered peptide ligand that we're going to be looking at is given by a subcutaneous injection, so it's given just under the skin. The way that the drug will be administered is with a weekly dose up front for five weeks and then it will shift over to just a once monthly dose. One of the things that's so exciting about this is that if it worked out, it's so much more convenient than some of the things we have right now.

How is this treatment different from standard treatment?

Dr. Thrower: We think that the altered peptide ligand would have several potential advantages. First would be that it's probably more specific in treating MS. We've really gone from an era pre-1993 of just suppressing the immune system or sort of taking a sledge hammer and beating the immune system into submission. Then in 1993, we had the first of a class of drugs called immune modulators, drugs that really fine-tuned the immune system and tried to tone things down. I think what the altered peptide ligand would represent is an even more specific way of doing that. Right now, all of our medications are given by injection ranging from once a week to every other day to one that's three times weekly, one that's given every day. The altered peptide ligand in this trial is going to be given weekly for the first five weeks, and then it would be given by subcutaneous injection once a month, so just from a convenience standpoint, it would represent a big improvement.

Why is this being considered a breakthrough?
Dr. Thrower: The altered peptide ligand I think would be considered a breakthrough because again, it's just another step forward in how specifically we can fine-tune the immune system in a person with multiple sclerosis. The other reason that it could be a breakthrough, and this may be further down the line in terms of getting information on this, is this pathway for working with the immune system has the possibility for being used outside of multiple sclerosis. There is a suggestion that when you modulate the immune system, you send the immune system toward it's more protective sort of white blood cell, that that more protective white blood cell may actually make some things in the brain and central nervous system that can lend these sorts of medications to being used outside of MS, things like Parkinson's disease or Lou Gehrig's disease. Again, we don't know that yet, and it's down the line, but we're starting to see the MS research overlap a lot with spinal cord research and research into neurodegenerative conditions like Parkinson's disease.

What were some of the benefits that you saw when using NBI-5788?
Dr. Thrower: The benefits that we saw from the earlier trials were that it appeared to be a well-tolerated mediation, it was easy to give in a once-

monthly dose, it suppressed the MRI activity, mainly in the form of active inflammation. The trials were not designed specifically to look at things like relapse rates and progression of disability, but that would be the hope also is that it doesn't just make the MRI look better, but that it actually slows down the clinical activity of someone's multiple sclerosis.

Copyright © 2003, Ivanhoe Broadcast News

Healthcare Professionals

Physical Therapist Interview-Bonnie

Interviewer: Okay, what I'm doing now is a little test; I'm going to start with the questions. There are only like 7 questions. This should record it. If I don't get a clear recording, I will call you....hehehe. But, it should work with no problem.

Interviewer: What made you decide to become a physical therapist?

Bonnie: I did a peer counseling, actually. By the time I got to Grad school for computer science, I realized that the career path I was going in was not what I really wanted to do and I couldn't see myself doing that for the rest of my life. So I went to career counseling and PT came up as a match for my personality and that made a lot of sense. And then ever since then, I just tried to get into PT school and finally got through it and made a turn into PT after about 5 years I finished everything. So, it just mad sense and I haven't questioned it since then.

Interviewer: How do your patients with MS differ from a regular patient? Say someone who has had a car accident?

Bonnie: They definitely have neurological symptoms that other patients do not have difficulty with balance and coordination. Um, and sensory issues as well. So, that's definitely a big difference. Also, fatigue is a big issue for patients with MS. You have to be aware of what the patient's limit is and make sure you are not fatiguing the patient with any activities that you do.

Interviewer: Yeah, that was a big thing. It's a very big thing.

Interviewer: What have you notice as a common physical problem with MS patients?

Bonnie: As far as outwardly, seeing people with MS?

Interviewer: Yes.

Bonnie: Um, It varies so much patient to patient. I don't think that you can say or visually tell someone has MS, just by seeing them sitting there. I mean, you really can't observe that It's more in the things that they do and the way that they are, able to coordinate their movements, those sorts of things sometimes you can see a difference. But just sitting or watching someone sitting, you couldn't tell off the bat that someone has MS.

Interviewer: For MS patients, what would you say is most important for them and maintaining mobility?

Bonnie: As far as what they need to do to maintain mobility. They just need to keep moving that is going to be the biggest thing for anyone who has a restriction in their mobility. Make sure that they are moving their limbs in all directions that they need to use them throughout the day and throughout their daily life. Just keep moving. That is really the biggest thing for that.

Interviewer: Yeah, because I remember (pauses and laughs). I used to try to dance all on the wrong beat and everything.

Bonnie: That's okay

Interviewer: (Laughs), but I was moving.

Bonnie: Exactly

Interviewer: So, that's why I did that. So, I guess that worked out. The next question is how can an MS patient help themselves at home to maintain mobility?

Bonnie: That's a good question, I guess get yourself into, oh you mean around the home?

Interviewer: Right.

Bonnie: Have a plan everyday to have a little bit of exercise or activity built into your day. Have some exercise set aside that you set aside time to do them every single day. That's probably the best thing. As far as modifications around the home for mobility, I guess someone needs to be able to,…I know you have the cane just to help you with walking around the home. Just make sure they are still able to walk with whatever aides they need around the home. Definitely keep those available. What other things exactly do you need?

Interviewer: Well, I know people use things like reachers and they use the thing, I don't know what it's called, but it helps you put your socks on and I can't think of the other thing, the hand thing and I can't think of what it's called.

<u>Bonnie:</u> The grabber, yes. Definitely any kind of assistive devices that you need to use to do what you can. I also think it's important to be able to do what you can and not rely on those pieces of equipment so much. If you absolutely need them, then use them, but actually using your hands and using your arms to do those activities will be the better thing, if you can. So, use what you can.

Interviewer: Right. Because, I have a reacher, but I rarely use it.

<u>Bonnie:</u> Good.

Interviewer: I will stand up on a step stool and stretch and get fussed at.

<u>Bonnie:</u> as long as you are keeping safe and not loosing your balance.

Interviewer: Well, apparently, I have a problem with the balance thing.

<u>Bonnie:</u> Yeah, that's the trade off. Actually, yeah.

Interviewer: (Laughs) I get fussed at a lot, but that's because I want to do it myself. I could ask someone else to do it for me, but...

<u>Bonnie:</u> You want to be independent.

Interviewer: Yeah, that's a big thing. Which is a good segway into the final questions, what as far as attitude, in dealing with MS patients is the best thing as far as helping them to cope with their situation?

<u>Bonnie:</u> Support groups, talking to other people who have been diagnosed. I know the question is a really big issue. As soon as you start loosing the ability to do the things you used to do is a downer and can get you down. But, I think having people around that you can talk to about what solutions they have used in their life to make their lives easier, um is huge. So, I definitely recommend that. Of course, coming to PT, I can always recommend that just to find out what you can do to keep yourself in the mood and keep yourself strong. Know your limits as far as your fatigue. I think that can definitely help with attitude and just knowing what your accomplishments can be, knowing what you are able to do. Just keep pushing that boundary. So, yeah, support groups. Huge.

Interviewer: Yeah, I like the support groups.

<u>Bonnie:</u> Have you ever been to any?

Interviewer: Oh, yes. As a matter of fact, when we were in South Carolina, I was there every month. I haven't gone to the one her as regularly because it's a greater distance and it's a conflict with scheduling since I can't drive like I used to. So, that's a problem for me. But, I get the newsletter and read them. I also call in. I am also on the volunteer list for the National MS Society, buddy program. So, I'm trying to work out some things and trying to give back as much as I can.

Bonnie: When were you diagnosed?

Interviewer: 1993. A long time ago. I have been living with MS most of my life, it seems to me. Because we can trace my symptoms back to when I was 10 years old.

Infusion Nurse-Wanda Bagley(2012 interview)

How long have you been working with MS patients? 7 yrs

What made you decide to work with MS patients? I love helping patients work through the challenges that MS can bring, and I LOVE to teach as well as learn. There is so much that goes on in the world of MS and research, and I get to teach and learn every day.

What have you noticed as a common problem with MS Patients? Fatigue and pain

For MS patients, what would you say is most important for them and maintaining mobility? COMPLIANCE!!! can't say that enough.

Would you say attitude and outlook on life play an important role for MS patients? Most definitely. Honestly the meds themselves can only do so much. I feel with MS and most diseases you need to have a "holistic" approach- healthy mind, healthy body/diet, healthy spirituality...

In your own words, tell me what you think about research, cures and MS. I find research to be both exciting and challenging at the same time. It's cool to see so many new treatments emerging and hopes of getting closer to a cure, but at the same time, the newer stronger drugs bring on more potential side effects- some of them detrimental, as well as not appropriate for all patients. Finding the right patient for the right clinical trial is a challenge in itself as well. But we keep hope alive :-)

If there was anything you could change for your patients, what would it be? If I could change anything it would definitely be the pain factor. It can be very difficult watching someone struggle with constant pain, and breaks my heart. Also, the financial struggle that a lot of MS patients have to go through is awful. I wish there was some way that treatment could be made more affordable to all.

Rakeeshia Dixon-Check-in (2012)

How long have you been working with MS patients? 4 Years

What made you decide to work with MS patients? My mother was dx with MS

What have you noticed as a common problem with MS Patients? Balance and Memory loss issues

For MS patients, what would you say is most important for them and maintaining mobility? N/A

Would you say attitude and outlook on life play an important role for MS patients? Yes

In your own words, tell me what you think about research, cures and MS. I think these studies are wonderful and I believe that one day they will find a cure for MS.

If there was anything you could change for your patients, what would it be? To have their abilities back..ect... memory balance ect.....To have a better outlook on life just remember you may have MS but it doesn't have you!!!!!

Erica Sutton- Clinical Research Coordinator (2012)

How long have you been working with MS patients?

I started working with MS patients in 1996.

What made you decide to work with MS patients?

When I started working on the Med Surg Unit as a (PCT) Patient Care Technician, the MS patients were apart of our assigned group. Back then, there weren't any outpatient IV rooms. The patients had to be admitted, for an extended hospital stay in order to receive their IV treatments.

What have you noticed as a common problem with MS Patients?

From my experience, fatigue, weakening of motor skills, cognitive function, vision, heat intolerance and ambulation all seem to negatively be affected, some mild, and others at a higher level of disability.

For MS patients, what would you say is most important for them and maintaining mobility?

As we all know it, in combination, Diet and Exercise is the "Universal Healer" to many of our medical, mental, physical, spiritual and emotional well beings. Many MS patients, have given rave reviews to low impact exercises, especially yoga because of it's ability to calm and balance ones over all body.

Would you say attitude and outlook on life play an important role for MS patients?
Attitude and outlook are the most important healing factors in anyone's health .A positive attitude offers higher altitude. We see it on a daily basis. The patients that come in with negative attitudes, are often the ones suffering with the most social and physical problems . Patients with more positive attitudes may suffer equally from the disease, but they seem to be less stressed and more willing to accept change and do whatever it takes. That type of attitude is often empowering for those that may be caring for or assisting that person with MS.

In your own words, tell me what you think about research, cures and MS.
 As a researcher currently running a spasticity trial for MS patients, I find that research is vital for this disease. I have worked on research projects were we are "searching for the cure" . In the meantime, our team is very focused on coordinating research projects with cutting edge therapies and treatments to improve the quality of life for MS patients.

If there was anything you could change for your patients, what would it be? Finding a cause and a cure!

Relapsing-Remitting MS

Most people living with MS usually have a type called relapsing-remitting. This generally begins in the 20's or 30's. The patient experiences periodic relapses, also called flare-ups or attacks. Once these are over then they have a period when the body may seem to be in remission or recovery. The disease does not get worse during these timeframes or breaks. These can be mild or severe. Hence the name relapsing-remitting MS.

MS is difficult for doctors to predict. I know scores of people with MS and none of us experience the same symptoms in the same way. A person's symptoms depend on where the MS plaques are in the central nervous system. A flare-up can last anywhere from 24 hours to several weeks. Multiple symptoms or just once (which can be new or an ongoing symptom) can flare-up.

Relapsing-Remitting MS Treatments

Relapsing-remitting treatments include medications, physical therapy and healthy habits. The sooner treatment begins, the better.

According to WebMD, some medications for relapsing-remitting MS fight the disease by turning down the body's immune system so that it doesn't attack nerves. These are called disease-modifying drugs. They may help keep the disease from getting worse for a while. They make the relapses less frequent and the symptoms less severe.

Here are the medications taken my injection:
1. Zinbryta (Daclizumab)
2. Copaxone (Glatiramer)
3. Avonex, Refib (Interferin beta-1a)
4. Betaseron (Interferon beta-1b)
5. Plegridy (Peginterferon beta-1a)

The following need to be taken at a clinic or hospital through an IV:

1. Lemtrada (Alemtuzumab)
2. Novantrone (Mitoxantrone)
3. Tysabri (Natalizumab)
4. Ocrevus (Ocrelizumab)

These can be taken by mouth as a pill:
1. Tecfidera (Dimethyl)
2. Gilenya (Fingolimod)
3. Aubagio (Teriflunomide)

There are side effects to these drugs. You and your doctor can talk and make a decision as to which one is best for you once her observes your symptoms.

Of course, the standard treat for an acute flare up is a round of steroids, either by mouth or IV. The steroids help reduce the inflammation in the central nervous system during an attack, as well as reduce the time and severity of the relapse. This is usually a high dose short-term course of steroids.

However, your doctor may prescribe other medications for different symptoms. These could include medications to fight fatigue, antidepressants or pain relievers.

A healthy weight and nutritious diet will also help fight the disease. Staying as active as possible for you and keeping a positive attitude made a big difference for me. I am not able to do much, but I walk at least a mile each sat. Of course, I do it in small increments so I do not tire my muscles to the point of fatigue. In addition, I don't want to get overheated. My physical therapist told me years ago that walking is a great way to get some exercise for me.

Resources

Shepherd Center
www.shepherd.org/

Shepherd Center is one of the top rehabilitation hospitals in the nation, specializing in medical treatment, research and rehabilitation for people with spinal cord injury or brain injury.

National Multiple Sclerosis Society
www.nmss.org/

The National MS Society is a collective of passionate individuals who want to do something about MS now—to move together toward a world free of multiple sclerosis. MS stops people from moving. We exist to make sure it doesn't.

Multiple Sclerosis Association
www.msaa.com/
MSAA is a national nonprofit organization whose mission is to enrich the quality of life for everyone affected by multiple sclerosis (MS).

Multiple Sclerosis Foundation
www.msfocus.org
The Multiple Sclerosis Foundation provides a comprehensive approach to helping people with MS maintain their health and well-being. We offer

programming and support to keep them self-sufficient and their homes safe, while our educational programs heighten public awareness and promote understanding about the disease.

MS International Federation
www.msif.org/en/resources/msif_resources/msif_publ ications/ms_in_focus/index.html

To lead the global MS movement to improve the quality of life of people affected by MS and to support better understanding and treatment of MS by facilitating international cooperation between MS societies, the international research community and other stakeholders through the following key priorities international research, development of new and existing societies, exchange of information and advocacy.

Consortium of MS Centers
www.mscare.org/
Mission-To be the preeminent professional organization for multiple sclerosis (MS) healthcare providers and researchers in North America, and a valued partner in the global MS community. Our core purpose is to maximize the ability of MS healthcare professionals to impact care of people who are affected by MS, thus improving their quality of life.

The Cleveland Clinic's Mellen Center for Multiple Sclerosis Treatment and Research

my.clevelandclinic.org/multiple_sclerosis_center/defa ult.aspx

They focus on addressing physical, emotional, cognitive and rehabilitation needs of the MS patient and their family members through a team approach.

Disability

Americans with Disabilities Act
www.ada.gov/

American Disability Association
www.adanet.org/

Mission:To meet the informational needs of Americans from Uruguay to Alaska with diverse disabilities. To promote awareness of disability culture by building bridges of understanding among all people. To enhance our collective quality of life and access to freedom.

World Institute on Disability
wid.org/about-wid
The mission of the World Institute on Disability (WID) in communities and nations worldwide is to eliminate barriers to full social integration and increase employment, economic security and health care for persons with disabilities. WID creates innovative programs and tools; conducts research, public education, training and advocacy campaigns; and provides technical assistance.

National Disability Rights Network
www.napas.org/
Mission: NDRN's mission is to promote the integrity and capacity of the P&A/CAP national network and

to advocate for the enactment and vigorous enforcement of laws protecting civil and human rights of people with disabilities.

The Council for Disability Rights

www.disabilityrights.org/

Mission: On national, state, and local levels, the Council for Disability Rights advances the rights of people with disabilities. The Council promotes public policy and legislation, public awareness through education, and provides information and referral services.

Social Security Disability Benefits

www.ssa.gov/pgm/disability.htm

The official site for the Social Security Administration

Disability World

www.disabled-world.com/

Disabled World provides a useful resource of information and news to the Disability Community, Organisations, and Rights Campaigners, via our Disability News Service, Articles, and informative Videos related to health and disabilities around the world.

Disability Resources on the net

www.disabilityresources.org/

Disability Resources, inc. is a nonprofit 501(c)(3) organization established to promote and improve awareness, availability and accessibility of information that can help people with disabilities live, learn, love, work and play independently.

Accessible Society
www.accessiblesociety.org/
The Center for an Accessible Society's goal is to focus public attention on disability and independent living issues. The project was funded by the National Institute on Disability and Rehabilitation Research from October 1999 through May 2004.

Disability.gov
www.disability.gov/
Disability.gov is an award-winning federal government website that provides an interactive, community-driven information network of disability-related programs, services, laws and benefits. Through the site, Americans with disabilities, their families, Veterans, educators, employers and many others are connected to thousands of resources from federal, state and local government agencies, educational institutions and non-profit organizations. New resources are added daily across 10 main subject areas – benefits, civil rights, community life, education, emergency preparedness, employment, health, housing, technology and transportation.

Disability Rights Advocates
www.dralegal.org/
DRA is a non-profit legal center whose mission is to ensure dignity, equality, and opportunity for people with all types of disabilities throughout the United States and worldwide.

The Institute on Independent Living
www.independentliving.org/
Mission: The Independent Living Institute (ILI) is a policy development center specializing in consumer-driven policies for disabled peoples' freedom of choice, self-determination, self-respect and dignity. Our ultimate goal is to promote disabled people's personal and political power. Towards this end we provide information, training materials and develop solutions for services for persons with extensive disabilities in Sweden and internationally. We are experts in designing and implementing direct payment schemes for personal assistance, mainstream taxi and assistive technology.

Employment

J.Lodge
www.jlodge.com
J.Lodge is the premier provider of contact center services in the world, bringing an unmatched level of service to your organization through our visionary database system, adherence to quality, and unmatched employee model. For over 11 years, J.Lodge has provided results driven feedback to our clients, allowing each to implement change that directly affects the bottom line.

Rat Race Rebellion
www.ratracerebellion.com
Our site will show you legitimate work at home jobs, home businesses, freelance projects, telecommuting friendly companies, and how to avoid internet scams.

NTI
www.nticentral.org/
NTI provides job opportunities for Americans with disabilities who require home-based work.

Enable America
www.enableamerica.org/index.html?gclid=CMndy-yprqkCFUff4AodvSwaLg
Enable America's objective is to increase employment among people with disabilities in the United States. To accomplish this goal, we are taking a two-pronged approach that reaches out to all

members of the disability community and the business community.

Federal Employment for people with Disabilities
www.opm.gov/disability/

Federal agencies fill jobs two ways, competitively and non-competitively. Persons with disabilities may apply for jobs filled either way. People who are selected for jobs must meet the qualification requirements for the jobs and be able to perform the essential duties of the jobs with or without reasonable accommodation.

Disaboomjobs
www.disaboomjobs.com/
You can search for jobs without registering, but if you do register, you can do all sorts of cool (and useful!) things. Not only can employers find you more easily, but you can save the information you find as you explore our more than 600,000 job postings.

Disability Jobsite.com
www.disabilityjobsite.com/
A career community for the Healthcare Industry. We provide new job openings for Disability Specialists every day, in addition to insightful research into the Healthcare & Medical employment market, and an informative career articles section, written and frequented by industry professionals.

Financial

Help Paying Medical Bills
www.needhelppayingbills.com/html/help_with_medi
cal_bills.html

The Assistance Fund
theassistancefund.org/
The Assistance Fund is a leading 501(c)3 nonprofit organization created to make advanced biotech therapies available to the underinsured. As new scientific discoveries are brought to market and diagnostics are created to establish appropriate therapy guidelines, The Assistance Fund works with individuals to make access a reality, putting us at the forefront of service delivery, speed to therapy and compliance to therapy.

Chronic Disease Fund
www.cd**fund**.org

Chronic Disease Fund® is a non-profit, full service financial and medication assistance organization. We exist to improve the health and quality of life of patients battling chronic disease, cancer or other life-altering conditions who cannot afford the medications they so desperately need.

Medication

Prescription Assistance
www.pparx.org
The Partnership for Prescription Assistance helps qualifying patients without prescription drug coverage get the medicines they need for free or nearly free.

RxAssist - Patient **Assistance** Programs
www.rxassist.org/
Patient assistance programs are run by pharmaceutical companies to provide free medications to people who cannot afford to buy their medicine. RxAssist offers a comprehensive database of these patient assistance programs, as well as practical tools, news, and articles so that health care professionals and patients can find the information they need. All in one place.

Prescription Drug Program, Patient **Assistance** Program, Free
freemedicineprogram.org/media.html
We, at Free Medicine Program, cut through the red tape by actually assisting you in applying for enrollment in patient assistance programs, and with the cooperation of your physician you may be able obtain prescription medicine free of charge.

Discount Prescription Cards
www.**discountprescriptioncards**.org/
You can save you an average of 15% to 20% on brand name drugs, and an average of 25% on generic drugs at over 58,000 pharmacies. These cards are supported   by pharmaceutical partners   who   have

negotiated lower rates on the prescriptions you need. There is NO charge for these discount prescription cards.

NeedyMeds
www.needymeds.org/

The mission of NeedyMeds is to make information about assistance programs available to low-income patients and their advocates at no cost. The NeedyMeds website is the face of the organization. Databases such as Patient Assistance Programs, Disease-Based Assistance, Free and Low- Clinics, government programs and other types of assistance programs are the crux of the free information offered online.

Pfizer medicines
www.PfizerHelpfulAnswers.com
Pfizer Helpful Answers is a family of assistance programs for people who have no insurance, or who do not have enough insurance and need help getting their Pfizer medicines.

Merck Programs to Help Those in Need
www.merck.com/merckhelps/

AstraZeneca: Patient & **Prescription Assistance** Programs
www.astrazeneca-us.com/help-affording-your-medicines/
Our commitment to improving health isn't just through our innovations in the lab; it's also through

knowing the people who use our medicines and helping them get these medicines when they need them.

Patient **Assistance** Programs - RxHope
www.rxhope.com/
RxHope is exactly what its name implies...a helping hand to people in need in obtaining critical medications that they would normally have trouble affording. We act as your advocate in making the patient assistance program journey easier and faster by supplying vital information and help.

Others

Assistive Technology - Independent Living Source - Amplified
www.iltsource.com/
Independent Living Source is dedicated to meeting all the assisted living technology needs of its consumers. It is a fact that more than 50 million Americans have some level of disability. ILS supplies this market with products that guarantee consumer safety, as well as the ability to go about their day without concern for injury. ILS's staff is well-educated on the products offered, thus passing this thorough knowledge to consumers.

Dmoz open directory
www.dmoz.org/Shopping/Health/Disabilities/Assistive_Technology/

National Accessible Apartment Clearinghouse

www.nmhc.org/Content/ContentList.cfm?NavID=182

My World of MS online community

This section has been developed to provide an online mutual support and Information forum. Registered users are given a greater level of interaction with other users, so that a true World of MS community may be created.

WebMD

www.webmd.com/multiple-sclerosis/news/20090428/high-doses-vitamin-d-cut-ms-relapses

Glossary of Common Terms

Abductor muscle
A muscle used to pull a body part away from the midline of the body (e.g., the abductor leg muscles are used to spread the legs).

Acetylcholine
Acetylcholine is a neurotransmitter. It is a chemical signal that transmits information from one nerve to another or from nerves to muscles.

Activities of daily living (ADLs)
Activities of daily living (ADLs) Activities of daily living include any daily activity a person performs for self-care (feeding, grooming, bathing, dressing), work, homemaking, and leisure. The ability to perform ADLs is often used as a measure of ability/disability in MS.

Acute
Having rapid onset, usually with recovery; not chronic or long lasting.

Adductor muscle
Adductor muscle a muscle that pulls inward toward the midline of the body (e.g., the adductor leg muscles are used to pull the legs together).

Adhesion molecules
Adhesion molecules are found on the surface of cells and help cells 'stick' together. They are important in

MS because they are involved in inflammation. At the sites of inflammation, cells lining the blood vessels produce adhesion molecules, which 'capture' passing white blood cells. The white blood cells are then able to enter the brain and attack myelin. Researchers hope that blocking the action of adhesion molecules will prove to be a useful treatment for MS.

Aetiology
Aetiology is the study of the causes of disease.

Affective release
Also called pseudo-bulbar affect; a condition in which episodes of laughing and/or crying occur with no apparent precipitating event. The person's actual mood may be unrelated to the emotion being expressed. This condition is thought to be caused by lesions in the limbic system, a group of brain structures involved in emotional feeling and expression.

Afferent pupillary defect
An abnormal reflex response to light that is a sign of nerve fiber damage due to optic neuritis. A pupil normally gets smaller when a light is shined either into that eye (direct response) or the other eye (indirect response). In an afferent pupillary defect (also called Marcus Gunn pupil), there is a relative decrease in the direct response. This is most clearly demonstrated by the "swinging flashlight test". When the flashlight is shined first into the abnormal eye, then in the healthy eye, and then again in the eye with

the pupillary defect, the affected pupil becomes larger rather than smaller.

Allele
An allele is one of the possible forms of a gene. For example, 'brown' and 'blue' are two alleles of the gene that affects eye color.

Amino acids
Amino acids are the building blocks of proteins. Hundreds or thousands of amino acids are combined to make a protein molecule.

Animal models
Animal models of diseases are the animal equivalent of human diseases. Researchers study animal models to better understand human disease and to try to find new treatments. EAE (experimental autoimmune encephalomyelitis) is an animal model of MS.

Ankle-foot orthosis (AFO)
An ankle-foot orthosis is a brace, usually plastic, that is worn on the lower leg and foot to support the ankle and correct foot drop. By holding the foot and ankle in the correct position, the AFO promotes correct heel-toe walking.

Antibodies
Proteins of the immune system that are soluble (dissolved) in blood serum or other body fluids and which are produced in response to bacteria, viruses, and other types of foreign antigens.

Antigen
Any substance that triggers the immune system to produce an antibody; generally refers to infectious or toxic substances

Assistive devices
Any tools that are designed, fabricated, and/or adapted to assist a person in performing a particular task, e.g., cane, walker, shower chair.

Ataxia
The incoordination and unsteadiness that results from the brain's failure to regulate the body's posture and the strength and direction of limb movements. Ataxia is most often caused by disease activity in the cerebellum.

Atrophy
A wasting or decrease in size of a part of the body because of disease or lack of use.

Autoimmune disease
A process in which the body's immune system causes illness by mistakenly attacking healthy cells, organs, or tissues in the body that are essential for good health. Multiple sclerosis is believed to be an autoimmune disease, along with systematic lupus erythematosus, rheumatoid arthritis, scleroderma, and many others. The precise origin and pathophysiologic processes of these diseases are unknown.

Autonomic nervous system

The part of the nervous system which regulates involuntary vital functions, including the activity of the cardiac (heart) muscle, smooth muscles (e.g. of the gut), and glands. The autonomic nervous system has two divisions: the sympathetic nervous system accelerates heart rate, constricts blood vessels, and raises blood pressure; the parasympathetic nervous system slows heart rate, increases intestinal and gland activity, and relaxes sphincter muscles.

Axon
The axon is the core nerve fiber extending from a cell body which is protected by the myelin sheath. It carries signals from a cell to another nerve cell or to a muscle.

Babinski reflex
A neurological sign in MS in which stroking the outside sole of the foot with a pointed object causes an upward (extensor) movement of the big toe rather than the normal (flexor) bunching and downward movement of the toes.

B-cell
A type of lymphocyte (white blood cell) manufactured in the bone marrow that makes antibodies.

Bell's palsy
A paralysis of the facial nerve (usually on one side of the face), which can occur as a consequence of MS, viral infection, or other infections. It has acute onset and can be transient or permanent.

Benign multiple sclerosis

Some people with multiple sclerosis are described as having a benign form of the disease. It is not possible to diagnose someone initially as having this form of MS, as it is only by looking at the disease ten or fifteen years after its onset that the pattern is visible. Benign multiple sclerosis has little impact on daily living. Individuals may experience a few mild attacks or relapses, but no ongoing disability.

Beta-interferon

The interferons are a group of signaling molecules in the immune system. Beta-interferon reduces inflammation. It has been licensed to treat people with relapsing-remitting MS and some people with secondary progressive MS (if they still continue to have relapses).

Blood-brain barrier (BBB)

A semi-permeable cell layer around blood vessels in the brain and spinal cord that prevents large molecules, immune cells, and potentially damaging substances and disease-causing organisms (e.g. viruses) from passing out of the blood stream into the central nervous system (brain and spinal cord). A break in the blood-brain barrier may underlie the disease process in MS.

Bone marrow

Bone marrow is the spongy tissue found in the middle of most bones. New red blood cells and some of the cells in the immune system are manufactured in the bone marrow.

Brainstem auditory evoked potentials (BAEPs)

A test in which the brain's electrical activity in response to auditory stimuli (e.g., clicking sounds) is recorded by an electroencephalograph and analyzed by computer. Demyelination results in a slowing of response time. This test is sometimes useful in the diagnosis of MS because it can confirm the presence of a suspected lesion or identify the presence of an unsuspected lesion that has produced no symptoms. BAEPs have been shown to be less useful in the diagnosis of MS than either visual or somatosensory evoked potentials.

Brain stem

The part of the central nervous system which houses the nerve centers of the head as well as the centers for respiration and heart control. It extends from the base of the brain to the spinal cord.

Capillary

Literally this means: as thin as a hair. The word is almost always used to describe a fine, small blood vessel

Catheter

A hollow, flexible tube, made of plastic or rubber, that can be inserted through the urinary opening into the bladder to drain excess urine that cannot be excreted normally.

Cell
The smallest unit of living structure in the body. Cells in the human body have many different functions and are highly evolved. However, they can all form proteins and amino acids

Central nervous system (CNS)
The central nervous system (CNS) consists of the brain and spinal cord, which control the main bodily functions.

Cerebellum
A part of the brain situated above the brainstem that controls balance and coordination of movement.

Cerebral hemispheres
The cerebral hemispheres are the visible halves of the brain, left and right.

Cerebrum
The large, upper part of the brain, which acts as a master control system and is responsible for initiating thought and motor activity.

Chronic
Of long duration, not acute; a term often used to describe a disease showing gradual worsening.

Chronic progressive MS (CPMS)
In most cases, people with multiple sclerosis will experience a relapsing/remitting form of the disease.

For some people, however, the symptoms will increase over time with no periods of remission (when there are fewer or no symptoms). The degree of progression and the time over which it takes place will vary from one person to another.

Clinical finding
An observation made during a medical examination indicating change or impairment in a physical or mental function

Clinical trial
Clinical trials are research studies involving patients, which compare a new or different type of treatment with the best treatment currently available. No matter how promising a new treatment may appear, it must go through a proper clinical trial before its benefits and risks can be certain.

Cognition
High level functions carried out by the human brain, including comprehension and use of speech, visual perception and construction, calculation ability, attention (information processing), memory, and executive functions such as planning, problem-solving, and self-monitoring.

Cognitive rehabilitation
Techniques designed to improve the functioning of individuals whose cognition is impaired because of physical trauma or disease. Rehabilitation strategies are designed to improve the impaired function via repetitive drills or practice, or to compensate impaired

functions that are not likely to improve. Cognitive rehabilitation is provided by psychologists and neuropsychologists, speech/language pathologists, and occupational therapists. While these three types of specialists use different assessment tools and treatment strategies, they share the common goal of improving the individual's ability to function as independently and safely as possible in the home and work environment.

Cognitive dysfunction
Cognitive dysfunction describes the problems that some people with MS have with thinking and remembering.

Cognitive function
The word cognitive is used to describe mental activities such as thinking, learning and remembering. Thus, somebody with normal cognitive function can perform these activities to a good standard

Cognitive impairment
Changes in cognitive function caused by trauma or disease process. Some degree of cognitive impairment occurs in approximately 50-60% of people with MS, with memory, information processing, and executive functions being the most commonly affected functions.

Combined (bladder) dysfunction
Combined (bladder) dysfunction A type of neurogenic bladder dysfunction is MS (also called detrusor-external sphincter dyssynergia - DESD).

Simultaneous contractions of the bladder's detrusor muscle and external sphincter cause urine to be trapped in the bladder, resulting in symptoms of urinary urgency, hesitancy, dribbling, and incontinence.

Computerized axial tomography (CAT scan)

A non-invasive diagnostic radiology technique for examining soft tissues of the body. A computer integrates X-ray scanned "slices" of the organ being examined into a cross-sectional picture.

Condom catheter

A tube connected to a thin, flexible sheath that is worn over the penis to allow drainage of urine into a collection system; can be used to manage male urinary incontinence.

Constipation

A condition in which bowel movements happen less frequently than is normal for the particular individual, or the stool is small, hard, and difficult or painful to pass.

Contraction

A shortening of muscle fibers that results in the movement of a joint.

Contracture

A permanent shortening of the muscles and tendons adjacent to a joint, which can result from severe, untreated spasticity and interferes with normal movement around the affected joint. If left untreated, the affected joint can become frozen in a flexed (bent) position.

Coordination
An organized working together of muscles and groups of muscles aimed at bringing about a purposeful movement such as walking or standing.

Cortex
The outer layer of gray matter that covers the surface of the cerebral hemisphere (brain tissue).

Corticosteroids
Steroids are naturally occurring hormones in the body. Corticosteroids are hormones produced by the adrenal gland in times of stress. They are effective in reducing inflammation. Synthetic versions of corticosteroids are used to treat relapses in MS.

Cortisone
A glucocorticoid steroid hormone produced either by the adrenal glands or synthetically, that has anti-inflammatory and immune-system suppressing properties. Prednisone and prednisolone also belong to this group of substances.

Cranial nerves
Nerves that carry sensory, motor, or parasympathetic fibers to the face and neck. Included among this group of twelve nerves are the optic nerve (vision), trigeminal nerve (sensation along the face), vagus

nerve (pharynx and vocal cords). Evaluation of cranial nerve function is part of the standard neurological exam.

Deep tendon reflexes
The involuntary jerks that are normally produced at certain spots on a limb when the tendons are tapped with a hammer. Reflexes are tested as part of the standard neurological exam.

Dementia
A generally profound and progressive loss of intellectual function, sometimes associated with personality change, that results from loss of brain substance, and is sufficient to interfere with a person's normal, functional activities.

Demyelination
A loss of myelin in the white matter of the central nervous system (brain, spinal cord).

Deoxyribose nucleic acid (DNA)
DNA is the genetic material found inside every living cell. It consists of two long chains of nucleotides twisted into a double helix and joined by hydrogen bonds between the complementary bases adenine and thymine or cytosine and guanine. The sequence of nucleotides determines individual hereditary characteristics.

Detrusor muscle
A muscle of the urinary bladder that contracts and causes the bladder to empty.

Diagnosis
Diagnosis is the process by which a person is identified as having multiple sclerosis. There is no one test to date which shows categorically that a person has MS. The most accurate test to date is the MRI scan. The main diagnostic techniques are outlined in MS The Disease.

Diagnostic criteria
The diagnostic criteria for MS are the clinical, laboratory and MRI findings that confirm that a person has MS.

Diplopia
Double vision, or the simultaneous awareness of two images of the same object, results from a failure of the two eyes to work in a coordinated fashion. Covering one eye will erase one of the images.

Disability
As defined by the World Health Organization, a disability (resulting from an impairment) is a restriction or lack of ability to perform an activity in the manner or within the range considered normal for a human being.

Disease-modifying therapies
Medications that, while not curing a disease, are able to reduce or change (modify) some of the symptoms. In MS, disease-modifying therapies such as interferon beta may reduce the frequency of relapses and delay the course of the disease

Double-blind clinical study
A study in which none of the participants, including experimental subjects, examining doctors, attending nurses, or any other research staff, know who is taking the test drug and who is taking a control or placebo agent. The purpose of this research design is to avoid inadvertent bias of the test results. In all studies, procedures are designed to "break the blind" if medical circumstances require it.

Dysarthria
Poorly articulated speech resulting from dysfunction of the muscles controlling speech, usually caused by damage to the central nervous system or a peripheral motor nerve. The content and meaning of the spoken works remain normal.

Dysesthesia
Distorted or unpleasant sensations experienced by a person when the skin is touched.

Dysmetria
A disturbance of coordination, caused by lesions in the cerebellum. A tendency to over- or underestimate the extent of motion needed to place an arm or leg in a certain position as, for example, in overreaching for an object

Dysphagia
Difficulty in swallowing. It is a neurological or neuromuscular symptom which may result in aspiration (whereby food or saliva enters the airway),

slow swallowing (possibly resulting in inadequate nutrition), or both.

Dysphonia

Disorders of voice quality (including poor pitch control, hoarseness, breathiness, and hypernasality) caused by spasticity, weakness, and incoordination of muscles in the mouth and throat.

Electroencephalography (EEG)

A diagnostic procedure that records, via electrodes attached to various areas of the person's head, electrical activity generated by brain cells.

Electromyography (EMG)

Electromyography is a diagnostic procedure that records muscle electrical potentials through a needle or small plate electrodes. The test can also measure the ability of peripheral nerves to conduct impulses.

Epidemiology

Epidemiology is the study of when, where and how a disease spreads through a population and how diseases can be controlled. It includes studies of the progress of disease and the experience of people with a chronic condition.

Euphoria

Unrealistic cheerfulness and optimism, accompanied by a lessening of critical faculties; generally considered to be a result of damage to the brain.

Evoked potential (EP)

EPs are recordings of the nervous system's electrical response to the stimulation of specific sensory pathways (e.g. visual, auditory, general sensory). In tests of evoked potentials, a person's recorded responses are displayed on a oscilloscope and analyzed on a computer which allows comparison with normal response times. Demyelination results in a slowing of response time. EPs can demonstrate lesions along specific nerve pathways whether or not the lesions are producing symptoms, thus making this test useful in confirming the diagnosis of MS.

Exacerbation (in MS)

The appearance of new symptoms or the aggravation of old ones, lasting at least 24 hours (synonymous with attack, replace, flare-up, or worsening); usually associated with inflammation and demyelination in the brain or spinal cord.

Expanded disability status scale (EDSS)

The EDSS is used to measure how disabled a person has become as a result of MS. It is one example of a number of different scales, which all measure slightly different things.

Experimental allergic encephalomyelitis (EAE)

Experimental allergic encephalomyelitis is an autoimmune disease resembling MS that has been induced in some genetically susceptible research animals. Before testing on humans, a potential treatment for MS may first be tested on laboratory animals with EAE in order to determine the treatment's efficacy and safety.

Extensor spasm
A symptom of spasticity in which the legs straighten suddenly into a stiff, extended position. These spasms, which typically last for several minutes, occur most commonly in bed at night or on rising from bed.

Fatigue
Fatigue is a feeling of overwhelming tiredness. It is a common symptom of MS, affecting 85% of people with the condition.

Fibroblast
Fibroblasts are found in connective tissue. This is the tissue that holds together the different structures of the body e.g. tendons and cartilage. Fibroblasts produce and maintain collagen - the main component of connective tissue.

Flaccid
A decrease in muscle tone resulting in weakened muscles and therefore loose, "floppy" limbs.

Flavonoids
Flavonoids are a widespread group containing over 4000 naturally occurring compounds, mainly found in fruit and vegetables, of which many are known to have anti-inflammatory, antiviral and anticarcinogenic properties. The anti-inflammatory

action of many, but not all flavonoids, appears to be largely based on their antioxidant effect.

Flexor spasm
Involuntary, sometimes painful contractions of the flexor muscles, which pull the legs upward into a clenched position. These spasms, which last two to three seconds, are symptoms of spasticity. They often occur during sleep, but can also occur when the person is in a seated position.

Food and Drug Administration (FDA)
The U.S. federal agency that is responsible for enforcing governmental regulations pertaining to the manufacture and sale of food, drugs, and cosmetics. Its role is to prevent the sale of impure or dangerous substances. Any new drug that is proposed for the treatment of MS must be approved by the FDA.

Foot drop
A condition of weakness in the muscles of the foot and ankle, caused by poor nerve conduction, which interferes with a person's ability to flex the ankle and walk with a normal heel-toe pattern. The toes touch the ground before the heel, causing the person to trip or lose balance.

Frontal lobes
The largest lobes of the brain. The anterior (front) part of each of the cerebral hemispheres that make up the cerebrum. The back part of the frontal lobe is the motor cortex, which controls voluntary movement; the area of the frontal lobe that is further forward is

concerned with learning, behavior, judgment, and personality.

Functional magnetic resonance imaging (fMRI)

fMRI is an imaging technique that can be used to detect brain activity. The technique measures blood flow to the brain. Highly active brain regions are detected because they require an increased supply of blood.

Gadolinium

A chemical compound that can be administered to a person during magnetic resonance imaging to help distinguish between new lesions and old lesions.

Gamma aminobutyric acid (GABA)

GABA is a neurotransmitter. It is a chemical signal that transmits information from one nerve to another.

Gastrocolic reflex

A mass peristaltic (coordinated, rhythmic, smooth muscle contraction that acts to force food through the digestive tract) movement of the colon that often occurs fifteen to thirty minutes after ingesting a meal.

Gene

DNA is the genetic material found in every cell. A gene is a stretch of DNA that includes all the information about how and when to make a specific protein. A cell will 'read' a particular gene every time it needs to make that protein. The proteins inside a cell determine what type of cell it is and what it can do.

Genetic susceptibility

With some conditions, e.g. cystic fibrosis, genetic factors make it certain that a person will eventually get a disease if they inherit certain genes. In other cases, genetic factors only make it more likely that a person will get a disease. This is true for MS. People who are genetically susceptible to MS also need to be exposed to one or more (as yet unknown) environmental factors before they develop the condition.

Glatiramer acetate

A synthetic drug made of amino acids used as a disease modifying therapy in MS

Glial cells

The central nervous system consists of neurons and glial cells. Neurons constitue about half the volume of the central nervous system and glial cells make up the rest. Glial cells provide support and protection for neurons. They are thus known as the "supporting cells" of the nervous system. The four main functions of glial cells are: to surround neurons and hold them in place, to supply nutrients and oxygen to neurons, to insulate one neuron from another, and to destroy and remove the carcasses of dead neurons (clean up). The three types of glia cells are: astrocytes, oligodendrocytes, and microglia.

Glucocorticoids
Glucocorticoids are a type of steroid hormone found naturally in the body. They affect carbohydrate metabolism, control the immune system and have an anti-inflammatory effect. A synthetic version is used to treat relapses in MS.

Glutamate
Glutamate is a neurotransmitter. It is a chemical signal that transmits information from one nerve to another.

Grey matter
Grey matter refers to the areas in the brain and spinal cord where nerves do not have a myelin sheath. These areas are darker in color.

Haematopoiesis
Haematopoiesis is the process of producing new red and white blood cells. It takes place in the bone marrow.

Handicap
As defined by the World Health Organization, a handicap is a disadvantage, resulting from an impairment or a disability, that interferes with a person's efforts to fulfill a role that is normal for that person. Handicap is therefore a social concept, representing the social and environmental

consequences of a person's impairments and disabilities.

Helper T-lymphocytes
White blood cells that are a major contributor to the immune system's inflammatory response against myelin.

Hemiparesis
Weakness of one side of the body, including one arm and one leg

Hemiplegia
Paralysis of one side of the body, including one arm and one leg

Herpes virus
There are a number of herpes viruses including the viruses that cause oral and genital herpes (HSV 1 and 2) and human herpes virus 6 (HHV-6). Some researchers believe HHV-6 may be linked to MS.

Human endogenous retrovirus (HERV)
HERVs are viruses that at some time in the past integrated themselves into human DNA. They are now passed on from one generation to the next. Some researchers believe they may be linked to MS.

Hyperbaric oxygen
A procedure in which the person breathes oxygen under greater than atmospheric pressure in a specially constructed chamber. Once thought to be a potential

treatment for MS, it has been evaluated in several controlled, double-blind studies and found to be ineffective for this purpose.

Immune response

The immune response refers to the activity of the immune system following infection or injury. A complex cascade of reactions takes place:

signalling molecules are released

local temperature is raised

blood vessels dilate and become more permeable

several different types of white blood cell are summoned to the site to remove the foreign body and/or repair the damage

Immune system

A complex system of various types of cells that protects the body against disease producing organisms and other foreign invaders. The immune system is made up of organs (e.g. lymph glands), specialised cells (white blood cells) and signaling molecules (e.g. antibodies). The immune system protects us from disease by recognizing and neutralizing any foreign matter in the body. It will:

destroy bacteria and viruses

neutralize toxins

repair damage to cells following injury

destroy the body's own cells if they are no longer functioning properly e.g. to prevent cancer

Immunoglobulin

Immunoglobulins are the proteins that form antibodies. Because antibodies regulate the immune system response, immunoglobulins are being researched as a treatment for MS

Immunology
This is the study of the immune system and how it works.

Immunosuppression
In MS, a form of treatment which slows or inhibits the body's natural immune responses, including those directed against the body's own tissues. Examples of immunosuppressive treatments in MS include cyclosporin, methotrexate, and azathioprine.

Impairment
As defined by the World Health Organization, an impairment is any loss or abnormality of psychological, physiological, or anatomical structure or function. It represents a deviation from the person's usual biomedical state. An impairment is thus any loss of function directly resulting from injury or disease.

Incidence
The number of new cases of a disease in a specified population over a defined period of time.

Incontinence
Also called spontaneous voiding; the inability to control passage of urine or bowel movements.

Indwelling catheter

A type of catheter (see Catheter) that remains in the bladder on a temporary or permanent basis. It is used only when intermittent catheterization is not possible or is medically contraindicated. The most common type of indwelling catheter is a Foley catheter, which consists of a flexible rubber tube that is inserted in the bladder to allow the urine to flow into an external drainage bag. A small balloon, inflated after insertion, holds the Foley catheter in place.

Inflammation
Inflammation describes the body's reaction to injury or infection. It is part of the immune response. Outside of the central nervous system (CNS) inflammation causes the blood supply to the area to be increased and large numbers of white blood cells to be released. Inside the CNS inflammation causes myelin damage. Active lesions in MS are sites of inflammation.

Intention tremor
Rhythmic shaking which occurs in the course of a purposeful movement, such as reaching to pick something up or bringing an outstretched finger in to touch one's nose.

Interferon
A group of immune system proteins, produced and released by cells infected by a virus, which inhibit viral multiplication and modify the body's immune response. One of the interferons, interferon beta-1b (Betaseron®) was approved by the Food and Drug Administration in 1993 for treatment of relapsing-

remitting MS. It was found in a clinical trial to reduce the frequency and severity of exacerbations by approximately 30 percent. A second interferon, interferon beta-1a (Avonex®) has also been shown to reduce the frequency and severity of MS exacerbations in people with relapsing-remitting disease. Avonex® was approved for use in MS in 1996.

Intermittent self-catheterization (ISC)
A procedure in which the person periodically inserts a catheter into the urinary opening to drain urine from the bladder. ISC is used in the management of bladder dysfunction to drain urine that remains after voiding, prevent bladder distention, prevent kidney damage, and restore bladder function.

Intramuscular (IM) injection
An injection given directly into the muscle of the body, such as the thigh or upper arm

Intravenous
Within a vein; often used in the context of an injection into a vein of medication dissolved in a liquid.

Lesion
In MS, lesions (or plaques) are patches in the central nervous system where inflammation has resulted in the loss of myelin. Some lesions will spontaneously repair themselves and disappear. Others become permanent areas of visible scarring.

L'Hermitte's sign
An abnormal sensation of electricity or "pins and needles" going down the spine into the arms and legs that occurs when the neck is bent forward so that the chin touches the chest.

License
Before a drug can be prescribed to a member of the public, it goes through an approval procedure to check that it is high quality, safe and effective. There may be a time lag between approval and launch; so a drug can be licensed but unavailable

Lumbar puncture
A diagnostic procedure that uses a hollow needle (canula) to penetrate the spinal canal at the level of third-fourth or fourth-fifth lumbar vertebrae to remove cerebrospinal fluid for analysis. This procedure is used to examine the cerebrospinal fluid for changes in composition that are characteristic of MS (e.g. elevated white cell count, elevated protein content, the presence of oligoclonal bands).

Lymph
Lymph is the fluid that flows through the lymphatic system. It transports white blood cells around the body to carry out an immune response wherever they are needed. The lymphatic system connects up with the blood vessels in the body. Together blood and lymph keep fluid circulating round the body.

Lymph nodes

Lymph nodes are small bean-shaped glands located throughout the body that form part of the immune system. White blood cells multiply in these nodes in preparation for an immune response. This is why lymph glands become swollen at the site of an infection.

Magnetic transfer imaging (MT)
MT is a new form MRI that has been used extensively in MS research. It is better at detecting damage to the brain than standard MRI

Magnetic Resonance Imaging (MRI)
A diagnostic procedure which produces visual images of different body parts without the use of X-rays. Nuclei of atoms are influenced by a high frequency electromagnetic impulse inside a strong magnetic field. The nuclei then give off resonating signals which can produce pictures of parts of the body. An important diagnostic tool in MS, MRI makes it possible to visualize and count lesions in the white matter of the brain and spinal cord.

Membrane
A thin layer of flexible tissue that separates or connects two structures or acts as a covering for a body part. For example, each cell in the body is enclosed in a membrane

Minimal Record of Disability (MRD)
A standardized method for quantifying the clinical status of a person with MS. The MRD is made up of five arts; demographic information; the Neurological

Functional Systems (developed by John Kurtzke) which assign scores to clinical findings for each of the various neurologic systems in the brain and spinal cord (pyramidal, cerebellar, brainstem, sensory, visual, mental, bowel and bladder); the Disability Status Scale(developed by John Kurtzke) which gives a single composite score for the person's disease; the Incapacity Status Scale which is an inventory of functional disabilities relating to activities of daily living; the Environmental Status Scale which provides an assessment of social handicap resulting from chronic illness. The MRD has two main functions; to assist doctors and other professionals in planning and coordinating the care of persons with MS and to provide a standardized means of recording repeated clinical evaluations of individuals for research purposes.

Molecule
A molecule is the smallest part of a substance that can possibly exist on its own and still have the properties of that substance. It is usually made of a group of atoms. e.g. a molecule of water is made up of two hydrogen atoms and one oxygen atom.

Multiple Sclerosis
Multiple sclerosis (literally, "many scars") is a disease of the central nervous system. The demyelination of the myelin sheath which coats the nerves impedes the transmission of signals from the brain. Most people diagnosed with multiple sclerosis will experience relapses in which the number of symptoms is increased. The main patterns which multiple sclerosis

takes are: relapsing/remitting; chronic progressive; secondary progressive; and benign.

Muscle tone

A characteristic of a muscle brought about by the constant flow of nerve stimuli to that muscle, which describes its resistance to stretching. Abnormal muscle tone can be defined as: hypertonus (increased muscle tone, as in spasticity); hypotonus (reduced muscle tone (flaccid paralysis); atony (loss of muscle tone). Muscle tone is evaluated as part of the standard neurological exam in MS.

Myelin

A soft, white coating of nerve fibers in the central nervous system, that is composed of lipids (fats) and protein. Myelin serves as insulation and as an aid to efficient nerve fiber conduction. When myelin is damaged in MS, nerve fiber conduction is faulty or absent. Impaired bodily functions or altered sensations associated with those demyelinated nerve fibers are identified as symptoms of MS in various parts of the body.

Myelin basic protein

Proteins associated with the myelin of the central nervous system that may be found in higher than normal concentrations in the cerebrospinal fluid of individuals with MS and other diseases that damage myelin.

Myelin sheath

The coating of the nerve fibers of the axon is referred to as the myelin sheath. This is made up of essential fatty acids which insulate the nerve fiber. During an attack of symptoms, or relapses, the sheath becomes inflamed, impeding the flow of signals from the brain. After the initial inflammation, the section of myelin sheath may become scarred, or demyelinated. The inflammation of the sheath does not always result in visible symptoms - so MRI assessments in clinical trials do not always relate to disability.

Myelitis
An inflammatory disease of the spinal cord. In transverse myelitis, the inflammation spreads across the tissue of the spinal cord, resulting in a loss of its normal function to transmit nerve impulses up and down, as though the spinal cord had been severed.

Myelogram
An X-ray procedure by which the spinal canal and the spinal cord can be visualized. It is performed in conjunction with a lumbar puncture and injection of a special X-ray contrast material into the spinal canal.

Natural killer cells
Natural killer cells make up 15% of white blood cells. They carry out one arm of the immune response, recognizing and destroying tumor cells or cells infected with a virus.

Nerve
A bundle of nerve fibers (axons). The fibers are either afferent - leading toward the brain and serving in the

perception of sensory stimuli of the skin, joints, muscles, and inner organs; or efferent - leading away from the brain and mediating contractions of muscles or organs.

Nerve block
A procedure used to relieve otherwise intractable spasticity, including painful flexor spasms. An injection of phenol into the affected nerve interferes with the function of that nerve for up to three months, potentially increasing a person's comfort and mobility.

Nervous system
Includes all of the neural structures in the body: the central nervous system consists of the brain, spinal cord, and optic nerves; the peripheral nervous system consists of the nerve roots, nerve plexi, and nerves throughout the body.

Neurologist
Physician who specializes in the diagnosis and treatment of conditions related to the nervous system.

Neurology
Study of the central, peripheral, and autonomic nervous system.

Neuron
The basic nerve cell of the nervous system. A neuron consists of a nucleus within a cell body and one or more processes (extensions) called dendrites and axons.

Neuropsychologist
A psychologist with specialized training in the evaluation of cognitive functions. Neuropsychologists use a battery of standardized tests to assess specific cognitive functions and identify areas of cognitive impairment. They also provide remediation for individuals with MS-related cognitive impairment.

Neurotransmitter
Neurotransmitters are chemical signals used to transmit information from one nerve to another or from a nerve to a muscle.

Neutralising antibodies
Over a period of time, an antibody may develop against protein based drugs (e.g., interferons) that limit their effectiveness. In these cases, some people with MS may experience a loss of the drug's effectiveness. However, the full implications of developing neutralizing antibodies are not yet fully understood

Nocturia
The need to urinate during the night.

Nystagmus
Rapid, involuntary movements of the eyes in the horizontal or, occasionally, the vertical direction.

Occupational therapist (OT)

Occupational therapists assess functioning in activities of everyday living, including dressing, bathing, grooming, meal preparation, writing, and driving, that are essential for independent living. In making treatment recommendations, the OT addresses: 1) fatigue management 2) upper body strength, movement, and coordination 3) adaptations to the home and work environment including both structural changes and specialized equipment for particular activities, and 4)compensatory strategies for impairments in thinking, sensation, or vision.

Oligodendrocyte
A type of cell in the central nervous system that is responsible for making and supporting myelin.

Optic atrophy
A wasting of the optic disc that results from partial or complete degeneration of optic nerve fibers and is associated with a loss of visual acuity.

Optic disc
The small blind spot on the surface of the retina where cells of the retina converge to form the optic nerve; the only part of the retina that is insensitive to light.

Optic neuritis
Inflammation or demyelination of the optic (visual) nerve with transient or permanent impairment of vision and occasionally pain.

Orthotic

Also called orthosis; a mechanical appliance such as a leg brace or splint that is specially designed to control, correct, or compensate for impaired limb function.

Orthotist
A person skilled in making mechanical appliances (orthotics) such as leg braces or splints that help to support limb function.

Paraparesis
A weakness, but not total paralysis, of the lower extremities (legs).

Paraplegia
Paralysis of both lower extremities (legs).

Paresis
Partial or incomplete paralysis of a part of the body.

Paresthesia
A spontaneously occurring sensation of burning, prickling, tingling, or creeping on the skin that may or may not be associated with any physical findings on neurological examination.

Paroxysmal symptom
Any one of several symptoms that have sudden onset, apparently in response to some kind of movement or sensory stimulation, last for a few moments, and then subside. Paroxysmal symptoms tend to occur frequently in those individuals who have them, and

follow a similar pattern from one episode to the next. Examples of paroxysmal symptoms include acute episodes of trigeminal neuralgia (sharp facial pain), tonic seizures (intense spasm of limb or limbs on one side of the body), dysarthria (slurred speech often accompanied by loss of balance and coordination), and various paresthesias (sensory disturbances ranging from tingling to severe pain).

Paroxysmal spasm
A sudden, uncontrolled limb contraction that occurs intermittently, lasts for a few moments, and then subsides.

Peptide
A peptide is a small protein. Proteins are made up amino acids. A peptide is made up of only a few amino acids, whereas a protein may be made of several hundred.

Percutaneous endoscopic gastrostomy (PEG)
A PEG is a tube inserted into the stomach through the abdominal wall to provide food or other nutrients when eating by mouth is not possible. The tube is inserted in a bedside procedure using an endoscope to guide the tube through a small abdominal incision. An endoscope is a lighted instrument that allows the doctor to see inside the stomach.

Peripheral nervous system

The peripheral nervous system is the collective name for the parts of the nervous system that are outside of the brain and spinal cord. It includes the nerves relaying information from the senses and the nerves that relay signals from the central nervous system out to the muscles.

Periventricular region
The area surrounding the four fluid-filled cavities within the brain. MS plaques are commonly found within this region.

Physiatrist
Physicians who specialize in physical medicine and rehabilitation of physical impairments.

Physical therapist (PT)
Physical therapists are trained to evaluate and improve movement and function of the body, with particular attention to physical mobility, balance, posture, fatigue, and pain. The physical therapy program typically involves (1) educating the person with MS about the physical problems caused by the disease, (2) designing an individualized exercise program to address the problems, and (3) enhancing mobility and energy conservation through the use of a variety of mobility aids and adaptive equipment.

Placebo
An inactive, non-drug compound that is designed to look just like the test drug. It is administered to control group subjects in double-blind clinical trials

(in which neither the researchers nor the subjects know who is getting the drug and who is getting the placebo) as a means of assessing the benefits and liabilities of the test drug taken by experimental group subjects.

Placebo effect
An apparently beneficial result of inactive therapy that occurs because of the patient's expectation that the therapy will help.

Plantar reflex
A reflex response obtained by drawing a pointed object along the outer border of the sole of the foot from the heel to the little toe. The normal flexor response is a bunching and downward movement of the toes. An upward movement of the big toe is called an extensor response, or Babinski reflex. This is a sensitive indicator of disease in the brain or spinal cord.

Plaque
An area of inflamed or demyelinated central nervous system tissue. In MS, plaque is an alternative name for a lesion.

Position sense
The ability to tell, with one's eyes closed, where fingers and toes are in space. Position sense is evaluated during the standard neurological ex am in MS.

Postural tremor

Rhythmic shaking that occurs when the muscles are tensed to hold an object or stay in a given position.

Post-void residual test (PVR)
The PVR test involves passing a catheter into the bladder following urination in order to drain and measure any urine that is left in the bladder after urination is completed. The PVR is a simple but effective technique for diagnosing bladder dysfunction in MS.

Power grading
A measurement of muscle strength used to evaluate weakness or paralysis. Power is tested as part of the standard neurological exam in MS.

Prevalence
The number of all new and existing cases of a disease in a defined population at a particular point in time.

Primary progressive MS (PPMS)
An alternative name for chronic progressive Multiple Sclerosis.

Prognosis
Prediction of the future course of the disease.

Prospective memory
The ability to remember an event or commitment planned for the future. Thus, a person who agrees to meet or call someone at a given time on the following day must be able to remember the appointment when

the time comes. People with MS-related memory impairment frequently report problems with this type of memory for upcoming appointments.

Proteins
Naturally occurring complex combinations of amino acids that are present in plant and animal cells and are essential to life. The human body contains over 100,000 proteins

Pseudo-exacerbation
A temporary aggravation of disease symptoms, resulting from an elevation in body temperature or other stressor (e.g. an infection, severe fatigue, constipation) that disappears once the stressor is removed. A pseudo-exacerbation involves symptom flare-up rather than new disease activity or progression.

Pyramidal tracts
Motor nerve pathways in the brain and spinal cord that connect nerve cells in the brain to the motor cells located in the cranial, thoracic, and lumbar parts of the spinal cord. Damage to these tracts causes spastic paralysis or weakness.

Peoria
The presence of pus in the urine, causing it to appear cloudy; indicative of bacterial infection in the urinary tract.

Quad cane

A cane that has a broad base on four short "feet," which provide extra stability.

Quadriplegia
The paralysis of both arms and both legs. Also called tetraplegia.

Randomised controlled trial (RCT)
An essential tool of medical research. An RCT is a study in which people are allocated (randomized) to different treatments and the effects of those treatments are compared. Some of these people may be randomized to a placebo or a standard treatment (the control), so that the effects of the test medication can be more clearly observed.

Recent memory
The ability to remember events, conversations, content of reading material or television programs from a short time ago, i.e., an hour or two ago or last night. People with MS-related memory impairment typically experience greatest difficulty remembering these types of things in the recent past.

Reflex
An involuntary response of the nervous system to a stimulus, such as the stretch reflex, which is elicited by tapping a tendon with a reflex hammer, resulting in a contraction. Increased, diminished, or absent reflexes can be indicative of neurologic damage, including MS, and are therefore tested as part of the standard neurological exam.

Relapse
Relapses are periods when people with MS experience new symptoms or when their old symptoms reoccur. Relapses can come on quite quickly, typically last for a few weeks, and vary from mild to severe. They may be followed by periods of remission, when the person with MS partially or completely recovers.

Relapsing/remitting MS (RRMS)
The pattern which multiple sclerosis follows differs for different people. The relapsing/remitting form of MS follows a course of relapses (also known as "attacks") where there is an increased level of symptoms, followed by remissions in which there are less, or no, evident symptoms. The periods of acute attack occur when the myelin sheath is inflamed, squeezing the nerve fibers so that messages do not pass clearly from the brain to other parts of the body. The frequency and severity of relapses varies. In a few cases, people with relapsing/remitting MS may go on to develop secondary progressive MS.

Remission
A lessening in the severity of symptoms or their temporary disappearance during the course of the illness.

Remote memory
The ability to remember people or events from the distant past. People with MS tend to experience few, if any, problems with their remote memory.

Remyelination
The repair of damaged myelin. Myelin repair occurs spontaneously in MS but very slowly. Research is currently under way to find a way to speed the healing process.

Residual urine
Urine that remains in the bladder following urination.

Ribonucleic acid (RNA)
RNA is a form of genetic material. It is produced when a gene is activated inside a cell. The RNA instructs the cell as to what proteins it needs to make.

Romberg's sign
The inability to maintain balance in a standing position with feet and legs drawn together and eyes closed.

Scanning speech
Abnormal speech characterized by staccato-like articulation that sounds clipped because the person unintentionally pauses between syllables and skips some of the sounds.

Schwann cells
Schwann cells are the cells that form myelin in the peripheral nervous system.

Sclerosis

Hardening of tissue. In MS, sclerosis is the body's replacement of lost myelin around CNS nerve cells with scar tissue.

Scotoma
A gap, blind spot or An area of diminished vision within the visual field.

Secondary progressive multiple sclerosis (SPMS)
In some instances, people who begin with a relapsing/remitting form of MS may find that over time the symptoms which they are experiencing increase. This may be a case of the remaining symptoms after each attack increasing over time, or the relapsing/remitting pattern may be replaced by a progressive pattern.

Sensory
Related to bodily sensations such as pain, smell, taste, temperature, vision, hearing, acceleration and position in space.

Sepsis
The presence of sufficient bacteria in the blood to cause illness.

Serotonin
Serotonin is a neurotransmitter. It is a chemical signal that transmits information from one nerve to another. Lowered levels of serotonin in the brain are linked to depression. Drugs like Prozac work by raising serotonin levels back to normal.

Sign

An objective physical problem or abnormality identified by the physician during the neurologic examination. Neurologic signs may differ significantly from the symptoms reported by the patient because they are identifiable only with specific tests and may cause no overt symptoms. Common neurologic signs in multiple sclerosis include altered eye movements and other changes in the appearance or function of the visual system; altered reflexes; weakness; spasticity; circumscribed sensory changes.

Somatosensory evoked potential

A test that measures the brain's electrical activity in response to repeated (mild) electrical stimulation of different parts of the body. Demyelination results in a slowing of response time. This test is useful in the diagnosis of MS because it can confirm the presence of a suspected lesion (area of demyelination) or identify the presence of an unsuspected lesion that has produced no symptoms.

Spasticity

The loss of normal elasticity in the muscles of the legs and/or arms as a result of disease in the central nervous system. It often results in extreme stiffness of the muscles.

Speech/language pathologist

Speech/language pathologists specialize in the diagnosis and treatment of speech and swallowing disorders. A person with MS may be referred to a speech/language pathologist for help with either one or both of these problems. Because of their expertise with speech and language difficulties, these specialists also provide cognitive remediation for individuals with cognitive impairment.

Sphincter
A circular band of muscle fibers that tightens or closes a natural opening of the body, such as the external anal sphincter, which closes the anus, and the internal and external urinary sphincters, which close the urinary canal.

Sphincterotomy
A surgical enlargement of the urinary sphincter in a male whose spasticity is so severe that he cannot empty his bladder. Once the surgery is performed, the man loses urinary control and must wear an external, condom catheter to collect the urine. This procedure is seldom required in MS. It is performed only on males because urinary drainage problems in females might lead to skin breakdown.

Spirometer
An instrument used to assess lung function; it measures the volume and flow rate of inhaled and exhaled air

Stance ataxia
An inability to stand upright due to disturbed coordination of the involved muscles, which results in swaying and a tendency to fall in one or another direction.

Stem cell
Stem cells are cells that can both reproduce themselves and develop into many different cell types. There is the potential to use stem cells to grow different types of cell on demand e.g. to grow new nerve cells. However, this research is still at the earliest stages. Researchers still don't know which chemical signals are needed to control cell growth.

Steroids
Steroids are natural hormones found in the body. They include the sex hormones, oestrogen and testosterone, and the corticosteroids that affect the metabolism and the immune system. Synthetic steroids are used to treat disease.

Subcutaneous (SC) injection
Using a needle to deliver medications into the tissue just under the skin

Symptom
A subjectively perceived problem or complaint reported by the patient. In multiple sclerosis, common symptoms include visual problems, fatigue, sensory changes, weakness or paralysis of limb, tremor, lack of coordination, poor balance, bladder or bowel changes, and psychological changes.

Synapse
The synapse is the connection between two nerve cells or between a nerve cell and a muscle cell. Nerve

signals are transmitted across the synapse by the release of chemical signals called neurotransmitters.

Tandem gait
A test of balance and coordination that involves alternately placing the heel of one foot directly against the toes of the other foot.

T-cell
A lymphocyte (white blood cell) that develops in the bone marrow, matures in the thymus, and works as part of the immune system in the body.

Tenotomy
An irreversible surgical procedure performed to cut severely contracted tendons attached to muscles that do not respond to any other type of spasticity control and are causing intractable pain and skin complications related to lack of physical movement.

Titubation
A form of tremor, resulting from demyelination in the cerebellum, that manifests itself primarily in the head and neck.

Tonic seizure
An intense spasm that lasts for a few minutes and affects one or both limbs on one side of the body. Like other types of paroxysmal symptoms in MS, these spasms occur abruptly and fairly frequently in those individuals who have them, and are similar

from one brief episode to the next. The attacks may be triggered by movement or occur spontaneously. See Paroxysmal symptom.

Transcutaneous electric nerve stimulation (TENS)

TENS is a nonaddictive and noninvasive method of pain control that applies electric impulses to nerve endings via electrodes that are attached to a stimulator by flexible wires and placed on the skin. The electric impulses block the transmission of pain signals to the brain.

Transurethral resection

A procedure to remove excess thickened tissue at the point of connection between the bladder and the urethra. This thickened tissue, which occasionally develops with the prolonged use of a Foley catheter, obstructs the flow of urine when the catheter is removed. This procedure is quite uncommon and is done mostly in males.

Transverse myelitis

An acute attack of inflammatory demyelination that involves both sides of the spinal cord. The spinal cord loses its ability to transmit nerve impulses up and down. Paralysis and numbness are experienced in the legs and trunk below the level of the inflammation.

Trigeminal neuralgia

Lightning-like, acute pain in the face caused by demyelination of nerve fibers at the site where the sensory (trigeminal) nerve root for that part of the face enters the brainstem.

Tumour necrosis factor (TNF)
TNF is a signaling molecule in the immune system. Because it is part of the mechanism causing inflammation, researchers are trying to find out if this molecule is important in MS.

Urethra
Duct or tube that drains the urinary bladder.

Urinary hesitancy
The inability to void urine spontaneously even though the urge to do so is present.

Urinary frequency
Urinary frequency describes the need to empty the bladder on a very regular basis. It is a common symptom of MS, caused by damage to the nerves associated with the bladder muscles.

Urinary urgency
The inability to postpone urination once the need to void has been felt.

Urine culture and sensitivity (C & S)
A diagnostic procedure to test for urinary tract infection and identify the appropriate treatment. Bacteria from a mid-stream urine sample is allowed to grow for three days in a laboratory medium and then tested for sensitivity to a variety of antibiotics.

Urologist
A physician who specializes in the branch of medicine (urology) concerned with the anatomy, physiology, disorders, and care of the male and female urinary tract, as well as the male genital tract.

Urology
A medical specialty that deals with disturbances of the urinary (male and female) and reproductive (male) organs.

Vertigo
A dizzying sensation of the environment spinning often accompanied by nausea and vomiting.

Vibration sense
The ability to feel vibrations against various parts of the body. Vibration sense is tested (with a tuning fork) as part of the sensory portion of the neurological exam.

Videofluoroscopy
A radiographic study of a person's swallowing mechanism that is recorded on videotape. Videofluoroscopy shows the physiology of the pharynx, the location of the swallowing difficulty, and confirms whether or not food particles or fluids are being aspirated into the airway.

Virus

A virus is a tiny microbe, much smaller than bacteria. Viruses cannot reproduce themselves and have to infect another cell to be able to do so. Viruses therefore enter cells in the body to cause diseases like flu, AIDS and chicken pox.

Visual acuity
Clarity of vision. Acuity is measured as a fraction of normal vision. 20/20 vision indicates an eye that sees at 20 feet what a normal eye should see at 20 feet; 20/400 vision indicates an eye that sees at 20 feet what a normal eye sees at 400 feet.

Visual evoked potential
A test in which the brain's electrical activity in response to visual stimuli (eg a flashing checkerboard) is recorded by an electroencephalograph and analyzed by computer. Demyelination results in a slowing of response time. Because this test is able to confirm the presence of a suspected brain lesion (area of demyelination) as well as identify the presence of an unsuspected lesion which has produced no symptoms, it is extremely useful in diagnosing MS. VEP's are abnormal in approximately 90% of people with MS.

Vocational rehabilitation (VR)
Vocational rehabilitation is a program of services designed to enable people with disabilities to become or remain employed. Originally mandated by the Rehabilitation Act of 1973, VR programs are carried out by individually created state agencies. In order to be eligible for VR, a person must have a physical or

mental disability that results in a substantial handicap to employment. VR programs typically involve evaluation of the disability and need for adaptive equipment or mobility aids, vocational guidance, training, job-placement, and follow-up.

White matter
The part of the brain that contains myelinated nerve fibers and appears white, in contrast to the cortex of the brain, which contains nerve cell bodies and appears gray.

What I've learned while living with MS

I can do anything I put my mind to. Determination and a positive attitude is half the battle. I fight my body everyday and each day that I can do the things I want to do, *I win*. I have MS, but MS does not have me. Push back, but don't overdo it. Learn your limitations and make your accomplishments within those boundaries. Do not let others steal your dreams with negative advice and words of limitations and doubt. Do the things that you love (as long as it is not dangerous). Laugh, smile and surround yourself with positive people and things. Have a strong support system. Don't be afraid to ask for help, but don't give up your independence. Realize that while MS is unpredictable, that having a sense of humor about things will make a big difference. Life with MS can be difficult, but it is not impossible.

So, back to my original question; what are bad nerves? Hmm, the simplest way to describe my bad nerves is bad electrical wiring. If the connection (cord) is broken or damaged, then the appliance or electrical equipment does not work properly, if at all. This is what happens in Multiple Sclerosis. So, just to be clear, my "bad nerves" is like "bad wiring". This explanation works for me without getting too technical since the disease is so complex and unpredictable. I hope this book will make it easier for others to understand and be able to explain the illness when   necessary.

About the Author

LJ Thomas is an author, show host, graphic designer and editor. She has lived with MS for over 20 years. During this time she and her husband have raised their two daughters. She has gotten and Associates and Bachelors and she is 2 classes away from her MBA.

LJ likes writing both fiction and nonfiction. She has a book on Domestic violence and a children's book (*Leo Learns About Anger*) series. She writes her fiction (*What Is This World Coming To?, Kidnapped in Love, Kidnapped in Love2: Backfire*) under Jamela.

LJ is an advocate against domestic violence and continues to work with authors. She hosts a show online called Purely Positive. The show spotlights positive people doing positive things for a positive community. At the printing of this book, the show is in it's second season. She believes anything worth having takes hard work.

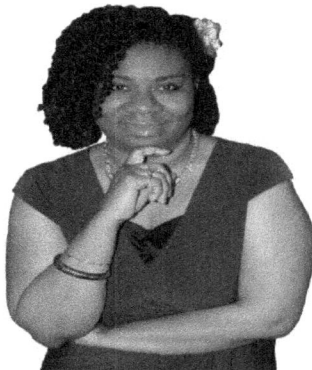

www.ingramcontent.com/pod-product-compliance
Lightning Source LLC
Chambersburg PA
CBHW060027210326
41520CB00009B/1035